CAMBRIDGE LIBRARY COLLECTION
Books of enduring scholarly value

History of Medicine

It is sobering to realise that as recently as the year in which On the Origin of Species was published, learned opinion was that diseases such as typhus and cholera were spread by a 'miasma', and suggestions that doctors should wash their hands before examining patients were greeted with mockery by the profession. The Cambridge Library Collection reissues milestone publications in the history of Western medicine as well as studies of other medical traditions. Its coverage ranges from Galen on anatomical procedures to Florence Nightingale's common-sense advice to nurses, and includes early research into genetics and mental health, colonial reports on tropical diseases, documents on public health and military medicine, and publications on spa culture and medicinal plants.

A Concise History of the Entire Abolition of Mechanical Restraint in the Treatment of the Insane

The most famous nineteenth-century British reformer of care for the mentally ill and disabled was undoubtedly John Conolly, whose 1856 *Treatment of the Insane without Mechanical Restraints* is also reissued in this series. However, Conolly's work at the Hanwell Asylum near London was based in part on the pioneering efforts of Edward Parker Charlesworth (1781–1853) and his younger colleague Robert Gardiner Hill (1811–78), who had already (and controversially) abolished physical restraint in the Lincoln Asylum by 1838. Conolly is known to have visited and been impressed by the Lincoln hospital, but his supporters, and his own book, suggested his primacy in the field, and Hill published this work in 1857 in order to refute Conolly's claims. The first part consists of Hill's account of his and Charlesworth's reforms at Lincoln, and the second reprints many of the letters and pamphlets which focused on the topic during this period.

Cambridge University Press has long been a pioneer in the reissuing of out-of-print titles from its own backlist, producing digital reprints of books that are still sought after by scholars and students but could not be reprinted economically using traditional technology. The Cambridge Library Collection extends this activity to a wider range of books which are still of importance to researchers and professionals, either for the source material they contain, or as landmarks in the history of their academic discipline.

Drawing from the world-renowned collections in the Cambridge University Library and other partner libraries, and guided by the advice of experts in each subject area, Cambridge University Press is using state-of-the-art scanning machines in its own Printing House to capture the content of each book selected for inclusion. The files are processed to give a consistently clear, crisp image, and the books finished to the high quality standard for which the Press is recognised around the world. The latest print-on-demand technology ensures that the books will remain available indefinitely, and that orders for single or multiple copies can quickly be supplied.

The Cambridge Library Collection brings back to life books of enduring scholarly value (including out-of-copyright works originally issued by other publishers) across a wide range of disciplines in the humanities and social sciences and in science and technology.

A Concise History of the Entire Abolition of Mechanical Restraint in the Treatment of the Insane

And of the Introduction, Success, and Final Triumph of the Non-Restraint System

ROBERT GARDINER HILL

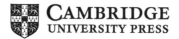

CAMBRIDGE
UNIVERSITY PRESS

CAMBRIDGE
UNIVERSITY PRESS

University Printing House, Cambridge, CB2 8BS, United Kingdom

Cambridge University Press is part of the University of Cambridge.
It furthers the University's mission by disseminating knowledge in the pursuit of
education, learning and research at the highest international levels of excellence.

www.cambridge.org
Information on this title: www.cambridge.org/9781108081740

© in this compilation Cambridge University Press 2015

This edition first published 1857
This digitally printed version 2015

ISBN 978-1-108-08174-0 Paperback

A CONCISE HISTORY

OF THE

Entire Abolition of Mechanical Restraint

IN THE

TREATMENT OF THE INSANE;

AND OF THE

INTRODUCTION, SUCCESS, AND FINAL TRIUMPH

OF THE

NON-RESTRAINT SYSTEM:

TOGETHER WITH

**A REPRINT OF A LECTURE DELIVERED ON THE SUBJECT
IN THE YEAR 1838;**

AND APPENDICES,

CONTAINING AN ACCOUNT OF THE CONTROVERSIES AND
CLAIMS CONNECTED THEREWITH.

BY

ROBERT GARDINER HILL, F.S.A.

MEMBER OF THE ROYAL COLLEGE OF SURGEONS, ENGLAND;
LATE ONE OF THE VISITORS OF THE LINCOLNSHIRE COUNTY LUNATIC ASYLUM;
AND FORMERLY RESIDENT MEDICAL SUPERINTENDENT OF THE LINCOLN
LUNATIC ASYLUM.

LONDON:
LONGMAN, BROWN, GREEN, AND LONGMANS,
PATERNOSTER ROW.
1857.

PREFACE.

—o—

In the following pages will be found a condensed but faithful statement of the origin and progress of the non-restraint system in lunacy, and the controversies connected with that origin. The system itself has triumphed over all opposition; and the claims of its Author have been universally acknowledged wherever the evidence of those claims has been accessible. The publication of the documents here brought forward seemed therefore only an act of duty, and the opportunity which it afforded for the expression of the Author's opinions upon important points connected with the judicious management of the insane, was not to be lost sight of. If the remarks here put forth shall tend in any degree to the amelioration of the condition of the insane, the object of the Author will be fully answered.

WYKE-HOUSE ASYLUM, and
INVERNESS LODGE, BRENTFORD.

—

May 4th, 1857.

CONTENTS.

—o—

and violent opposition of the *Lancet,* of Nov. 5th, 1853.
Refusal of the Editor of the *Lancet* to insert the
Author's replies.—Opinions of the *Stamford Mercury,*
(local County paper,) and of the Editor of the *Medical
Circular.* — Letters of Drs Wingett and H. van
Leeuwen.

Appendix (F.)—Testimony of the *Lancet* from 1840 to 1852,
in favour of the Author's claims.—Testimony of Richard
Mason, Esq., late Town Clerk of Lincoln, and a Governor of the Lincoln Lunatic Asylum.

Appendix (G.)—Cases of the two patients under treatment
at the Lincoln Lunatic Asylum during the period of
the Mitigation System, referred to in the historical
sketch.

HISTORICAL SKETCH.

HISTORICAL   SKETCH,

&c. &c.

TWENTY-ONE years have elapsed since I "expressed
my own belief, founded on experience in the Lincoln
Lunatic Asylum, that *it might be possible to conduct
an Institution for the insane, without having recourse
to the employment of any instruments of restraint
whatever;* "* twenty years have elapsed since I carried
out at that asylum what I had before conceived
possible; and eighteen years since I gave to the
world my published lecture on non-restraint, which
had been delivered about two years previously at
one of the public institutions of the city of Lincoln.
Subsequent events have shown that I was right in
my opinion; and the system has proved, as I
predicted it would, a blessing to the insane.†

---

* See the Thirteenth Report of the Lincoln Lunatic Asylum.

† " The annual reports presented by the resident physician in 1839,
1840, and 1841, contained the details of a plan adopted by him from the
Lincoln Asylum, and persevered in, with such modifications as
experience suggested, with the sanction of the visiting justices, to
dispense, in the treatment of the insane, with all the ancient bodily
restraints. The difficulties attending the commencement of the under-

In the lecture referred to, I affirmed that, in a properly constructed building, with a sufficient number of suitable attendants, restraint was not only unnecessary, but that it was *in all cases* injurious, and its application consequently unjustifiable. I have no doubt that almost all who were engaged in the treatment of the insane considered that declaration as absurd and impossible, as it was then novel and startling; but it must be borne in mind, that it was not made until I had for a long period actually lived amongst the patients for several hours daily, taking the duties of an attendant as well as that of House-Surgeon. I had therefore a full opportunity of judging whether restraint was, or was not necessary. I was satisfied that it was not : and although the statement might at first appear a very bold one, nevertheless it was my firm conviction that, under the conditions stated, the entire abolition of mechanical restraint was both practicable and humane; and I had no hesitation in staking my reputation upon it. Public attention was soon aroused, as well it might

---

taking, its progress, and its eventual success, have been already related in those reports without disguise, and it is believed, without exaggeration. The resident physician has now but the agreeable task of recording that time, and patience, and the zealous co-operation of all the officers of the asylum, have enabled him to overcome many obstacles, and have confirmed him in a belief, at first encouraged with much diffidence, but now established beyond the likelihood of ever being overthrown, that the management of a large asylum is not only practicable without the application of bodily coercion to the patients, but that, *after the total disuse of such a method of control, the whole character of an asylum undergoes a gradual and beneficial change.*"— Dr Conolly's Fourth Report of the Hanwell Asylum. 1842.

be, to the subject : for notwithstanding the bold efforts
of Pinel, and Esquirol, abroad, and the humane system
of the Retreat, and some other institutions* in this
country, no such statement as mine had been made by
any man living : neither had it ever been conceived
possible that mechanical restraint could be dispensed
with *in all cases*. Indeed for many years I was
stigmatised as one bereft of reason myself, a speculator,
peculator, and a practical breaker of the sixth commandment by exposing the lives of the attendants
to the fury of the patients. The system was called
" a piece of contemptible quackery, a mere bait for
the public ear." As regards the Lincoln Asylum, it
was most extraordinary, that notwithstanding the many
expedients previously resorted to with the avowed

---

* The Suffolk Asylum, *e.g.* in which, according to the statement of
Dr Kirkman, mechanical restraint was only resorted to in extreme
cases, although the principle of its entire abolition was not acknowledged, even after it had been adopted in other asylums ; neither I
believe does Dr Kirkman yet acknowledge it. In his report of
1840, Dr Kirkman says, " All personal confinement is invariably
removed on the entrance at the gate, and it is *very rarely* indeed had
recourse to again, even for an hour. *Whenever it becomes really
necessary, as in the case of the determined suicide*, at night, it is of the
gentlest possible kind that an effective guard can be."

It is clear, therefore, that in 1840 (and the two following reports
show that in the two following years restraints continued to be occasionally employed) Dr Kirkman did not consider that in the treatment of his patients mechanical restraints could in all cases be dispensed with.

How the doctor can reconcile this statement of his, with that which
he made in 1854, in answer to the inquiries of the Commissioners, viz.,
that " all instruments of mechanical restraint were destroyed more
than *twenty* years ago, and they have neither been used nor required
ever since," I am at a loss to imagine.

purpose of diminishing the number of restraints, so
great was the opposition, both within and without
the institution, that despite the constant and strenuous
support of Dr Charlesworth, I was ultimately compelled
to resign my appointment. In fact, it was impossible
to remain. The attendants were encouraged in acts
of disobedience, and all control was lost. Had I
retained my appointment, I must have sacrificed my
principles—and this alone is a proof that the abolition
of restraint was a thing never contemplated. The
proceedings at that time convinced me that the hire
and discharge of servants ought always to be in the
hands of the superintendent, and that the matron
also ought to be under his control: in fact, that the
resident superintendent should be the sole head of the
establishment, responsible of course to the proper
authorities.

The war against the system was for some time
confined to the Lincoln Asylum, and parties connected
with it ; but at length it assumed a more general
character ; and those who became converts to the non-
restraint system were in their turn the subjects of
virulent and abusive attacks. The first person who
adopted the system in its full extent was the late Dr
T. O. Pritchard, of the Northampton Asylum. He
carried it out in that institution soon after its opening.
Dr Pritchard wrote some excellent reports on the
management of that asylum. I had the pleasure of
his acquaintance, and had many opportunities of
observing the satisfactory way in which he and Mrs
Pritchard conducted the institution. I was present at

one of their balls given for the amusement of the patients, when the galleries were decorated with evergreens and flowers, and well lighted, and the patients, both male and female, enjoyed themselves much. It was extremely gratifying, in those early days of non-restraint, to see the good conduct and respectful demeanour of the patients, both male and female, when thus associated together. Such scenes are not now uncommon.

Before I take leave of Dr Pritchard, I must crave the liberty of transcribing the following extract from the Fourth Annual Report of the Northampton General Lunatic Asylum, pp. 65-6:

" Mechanical coercion. The practice of this hospital is too generally known, and too firmly established, to require many observations. It may, however, be excusable to give expression to the heartfelt satisfaction with which we review the early introduction of the 'humane system' to our institution. I have before reported that the experiment was unpremeditated; it did not arise from any preconception that physical restraint could be *totally* dispensed with in the treatment of the insane, though a strong feeling existed. that it had long been very unnecessarily and cruelly employed; but it was self-evident that an accurate estimate of the character and disposition of our patients, must precede any successful attempt to prescribe their moral management; and it was equally obvious, that this end never could be attained, so long as they were subject to the influence of those extraneous sources of irritation, which we confidently believed had contributed the most exaggerated and repulsive features of their distressing malady. The instant liberation, therefore, of every individual brought to the asylum in a state of coercion, was the natural consequence of these opinions, and the results of the trial were in the highest degree satisfactory. But though an insight was thus obtained into the latent powers of purely moral influences, I was indebted to the annual reports of the Lincoln Asylum, kindly forwarded by Dr Charlesworth, for the suggestion, that mechanical agency might be absolutely discarded. Many difficulties and apparent dangers, however, interposed to check our adoption of Mr R. G. Hill's system: an unfinished building, numerous workmen employed in every direction, the inexperience and timidity of the attendants—few in number, in consequence of a prevalent disinclination to enter into our service—all contributed, during the first year, to add to the anxieties of direction, and thwart my intentions, as well as to excite occasional doubts of their practicability. These impediments have long been surmounted, for they but stimulated renewed exertions and more extended inquiry; and we have now the gratification of knowing that similar results have rewarded the labours of a majority of the superintendents of the largest and most celebrated hospitals in the kingdom; and that unanimity of opinion on this vital question is rapidly pervading not only our own country, but also the great continents of Europe and America."

Next, after Dr Pritchard, came that "great and good man," Dr Conolly; and perhaps, but for him, the system might have been strangled in its birth. It was ordained otherwise. Mr Serjeant Adams, whose atten- tion had been directed to the new system at Lincoln, was in the habit of visiting the Lincoln Asylum when on circuit, and the result was, that when Dr Conolly received the appointment of physician to the Hanwell Asylum, Mr Serjeant Adams, who was one of the visit- ing justices at Hanwell, recommended Dr Conolly to visit Lincoln. Dr Conolly did so, and was so pleased with the quiet and order which he observed there, that on his return to Hanwell, he set to work vigorously with a view to abolish restraint in that giant establish- ment. Dr Conolly had many difficulties to contend with—difficulties similar to those experienced by myself at Lincoln—but he had the support of the committee. Dr Conolly was subjected to a very unwarrantable and unfounded attack by one of his colleagues, and was much harassed and annoyed; but, in spite of oppo- sition and insult, he succeeded. The following is a copy of the entry made by Dr Conolly on his visit to the Lincoln Asylum :—

" Having read Mr Hill's lecture, and the extracts from the minutes and tables in the Appendix, we visited this asylum with feelings of unusual curiosity and interest; and we have been deeply impressed with the *tranquillity*, as well as the general order and com- fort, pervading the whole establishment, all the arrange- ments of which have excited our admiration in a very high degree.

" J. Conolly, M.D.

" May 17th, 1839."   " W. Conolly, M.D.

I must be permitted to record here the able advocacy and defence of the system in the 'Lancet,' by the late Mr Serjeant Adams, as "Looker-on." He was, indeed, a most powerful advocate, and contributed greatly towards the support of the system in the days of its greatest trial.

Neither must I omit to mention the constant and unflinching advocacy of the 'Lancet' itself, which, beyond doubt, induced many of our public institutions to make a trial, more or less, of the effects of the new system. It was the medium of several communications from myself on the subject, and also of the defensive replies which I was obliged almost continually to make to various attacks upon the system, and upon myself as the author of it. During all this period I received the invariable support of that journal, which nevertheless afterwards surpassed the bitterest of my opponents in the envenomed malignity of its sarcastic abuse.

The triumph of the system, however, was now at hand. It seemed as if a new and blessed light broke in at once upon our asylums, and the doom of restraint and terror was pronounced. The large asylum near Glasgow was built, with all suitable arrangements, expressly adapted to the requirements of the non-restraint system; and, one by one, almost all our large asylums have since adopted it. In England alone about 14,000 lunatics are treated on its principles. "The gradual advance of the new system has, perhaps, been marked by no circumstance more striking than by that of the opening of at least ten English county asylums, of considerable size, within the last few years, without any preparation being considered necessary or desirable, in any one of them, for any application of mechanical restraints."* At first the Commissioners in Lunacy were not favourable to non-restraint, but for several years past they have done their utmost to promote it; and, to their honour be it recorded, they have caused several patients to be removed from asylums where they were kept in close confinement, to other institutions, where they can have the free use of their limbs, and the benefit of fresh air and exercise. The change has in almost every instance been attended with good effects, and sometimes with speedy recovery.

Thus, within a period of a very few years after its introduction, the non-restraint system had become, with few exceptions, the system of treatment throughout Great Britain : it had been adopted in some of the most eminent institutions of the Continent, and in America; and, even where not adopted, its merits were canvassed in a very different spirit from that with which they were first received. The noble efforts of that truly great and philosophical man, Dr H. Van Leeuwen, late physician of the Meerenberg Lunatic Asylum, Holland, contributed more than anything to pave the way for the introduction of non-restraint into the institutions abroad, and it is with the greatest pleasure that I embrace this opportunity of recording my unbounded esteem for his

---

* See 'The Treatment of the Insane without Mechanical Restraint. By J. Conolly, M.D.

enlightened character, and unwearied exertions in the cause of humanity.

It is to be deplored that so great a boon as the non-restraint system was to mankind should have occasioned so much controversy and so much bitter animosity. Such, however, having been actually the case, a sketch of the introduction of that system would be both incomplete and unfaithful if it did not contain some account of those controversies. The publication of them will throw much light on a subject concerning which the public have at present no complete and full historical account; nor indeed any to which they can refer for a connected series of documentary evidence.

And here, in entering upon this part of my narrative, I feel bound, in justice to myself, to state unreservedly that I never attacked any other institution, or any person holding different views from myself; that I never obtruded myself upon the public notice, except when compelled in self-defence by the virulent attacks made upon the system, or upon myself, or both; and that I never wished or attempted to derogate from the just claims of others, my predecessors, or cotemporaries, for their humane exertions in behalf of the insane, or for the improvement or modification of the existing mode of treatment. All I ever did, and that only when compelled to speak in self-defence, was to vindicate my just claim. (I hope with calmness and candour) to what was certainly never before either attempted or even contemplated, viz., the entire abolition of mechanical restraint in all cases of lunacy whatever, and the introduction of a system in which such restraint had no place.

There were two distinct periods and phases of the controversial attacks:—

1st. The attacks upon the system, and upon myself, as the author of it; which commenced almost immediately upon its introduction, and continued until the system, by its beneficial results and complete success, triumphantly vindicated its own merits, and bore down all opposition:—and

2ndly. The attacks which were made, *after the practicability and value of the system had been fully established by experiment*, upon my own claims to be its author. We will speak of each in their turn.

I. It was not unnatural,—it was to be expected,— that on the introduction of a plan of treatment, so thoroughly contrary to generally received principles, the merits of such a plan, and its practicability, should be extensively canvassed; and opinions, variously modified according to the views of the different writers, should be freely given on the subject. This was both natural and right, and in many instances was done in the most liberal and philosophical spirit: with a generous candour that cannot be too highly acknowledged, they were ready to give the new plan a fair trial, although they could not bring themselves to believe the possibility of its adoption with safety. Others attacked the system with a virulence which must ever be deplored, when connected with discoveries of such importance to the world.

The first public attack of this nature, unconnected

with the Lincoln Asylum itself, was made by Dr Corsellis, the medical superintendent of the West Riding Lunatic Asylum, Wakefield. In the report of that institution for the year 1839, Dr Corsellis makes the following remarks:—

" No one is placed under restraint but by the immediate order of the director, and as soon as the symptoms warrant their liberation all restraint is removed; many instances have, however, been known of patients who, feeling a return of excitement, have themselves requested to be again restrained; a proof that when they could exercise a judgment, they were sensible how beneficial restraint had been to them.

" To permit patients in a high state of excitement to keep up that excitement by constant muscular action, or knowingly to risk the lives of both patients and servants, would be treatment having no more of humanity in it than the name; and it requires but little practical acquaintance with the subject at once to detect its absurdity.

" The result of many years' careful attention to this subject had led to the conviction that a mild and judicious restraint can never be supplied by any *surveillance*. The presence of any individual is of itself sufficient, in many instances, to keep up the excitement; for it is a truth but too general that maniacs regard all around them as enemies, and exhaust themselves in vociferation, and attempts at violence; whilst force on the one part, and resistance on the other, keep up the unequal contest, ending sometimes in bruises or broken limbs."

The 'Lancet,' in commenting upon this report, Feb. 8th, 1840, says, "Dr Corsellis is somewhat at variance with the physicians of the Lincoln Asylum, and Dr Conolly, on the subject of restraint. We extract his observations, for we wish to lay all the facts before our readers, and to see the subject fully discussed. Has Dr Corsellis tried the system of surveillance fairly, for any time, or to any extent?"

Thus invited, as it were, by the Editor, I published the following letter on the results of non-restraint at Lincoln.

"TO THE EDITOR OF THE 'LANCET.'

"SIR,—In your last number I find an article on the 'treatment of the insane,' at variance with the views which I have advocated, and to the best of my power *will* advocate, respecting 'restraint' as applied to the insane. Can you spare a short space for the insertion of a few observations connected with this subject. The result of the non-restraint system at Lincoln Asylum has been, that

"1. All *recent* cases have been discharged recovered.

"2. Several cases considered to be *incurable* have been discharged recovered.

"3. The inmates are much more happy and comfortable than under the old system.

"4. Even the refractory ward preserves (in general) an orderly and comparatively quiet appearance; there has been a *marked increase* in the tranquillity of the establishment; 'the patients move about less, and talk less to visitors, than in any other Asylum which is known to us.'*

---

* 'British and Foreign Medical Review,' for Jan. 1840, p. 145.

" 5. Outbreaks and sallies of passion occur very seldom; fits of phrensy are of much shorter duration.

" 6. Many patients, insensible to the calls of nature, through previous restraint, have been restored to habits of cleanliness, who would otherwise have remained dirty and incurable.

" 7. No serious accident has occurred under our system of *surveillance*.

" 8. Lastly, no suicides have happened; no patients have been found dead in bed.

" There will be a prejudice against every improvement in science or practice at first, so long as it wears the appearance of an innovation upon long-established habits; but can these things be said of any asylum where restraint is kept up? Does restraint prevent accidents? Experience proves the contrary. Does restraint prevent suicide? Experience proves the contrary. Can a patient, insensible to the calls of nature, be restored to habits of cleanliness whilst under restraint? He cannot. Does restraint contribute to the recovery of the patient? Experience proves the contrary. It exasperates the sufferer, excites in him a spirit of revenge against the attendants, and thus is the fertile cause of accidents or injuries in an asylum. Lives are not risked by allowing maniacs the free use of their limbs; no accident, no suicide, has occurred since the adoption of this system at Lincoln. ' The insane are especially acute in discovering the exact capabilities of their attendants.'* An insane person is well aware

* The 21st report of the Director of the West Riding of York Pauper Lunatic Asylum, p. 5.

that he is not able to compete with three powerful attendants; hence, no force is required with *surveillance*; it is only necessary in *restraining* patients, for then they will do all in their power to prevent the instruments of restraint being applied. It is such contests that end in bruises and broken limbs. A keeper is insulted, perhaps only verbally so; the patient, instead of being soothed, is threatened, and the insult is repeated; a strait-waistcoat is brought, a struggle ensues, another keeper arrives, and in the attempt to put on the jacket the patient gets very roughly used. He resists, swears, kicks, and bites; the keeper or keepers kneel upon his body, thrust their knuckles into his throat, beat him and bruise him, until they succeed in overcoming him. Then the jacket is tied so tightly that he can scarcely breathe; his legs are fastened together, either with iron or leathern hobbles; and, to sum up all, if he have resisted stoutly, he is chained to a wall in a small dark room, and the door is closed upon him. This having occurred, the attendant goes to his master's room, informs him that such a patient has been violent, &c., and that he was compelled to restrain him. The superintendent visits him; he has an opportunity then (suppose) of complaining of such usage. The reply he obtains is, that had he conducted himself properly the keeper would have had no occasion to restrain him. At bed-time, instead of being allowed to go to his proper bed, he is thrown upon straw, and his hands and feet are chained to the bedstead. How long he remains so is now a problem. The keeper thinks it would be dangerous to liberate him; this is sufficient; his fate is sealed. The poor unfortunate sufferer becomes insensible to the calls of nature, not having it in his power to assist himself. For weeks, months, perhaps years, he wallows in his filth; imbecility or idiotcy follows ; his health and strength gradually sink, and the attendant, some morning, on opening the door of his cell, finds that he has ceased to exist.

" Such is a faithful picture of what has frequently occurred, and must occur, under the system of restraint. Restraint, too, not muscular action, keeps up excitement. If a patient be allowed his liberty whilst under excitement, he soon exhausts himself.

" To conclude these observations, non-restraint is practicable, for we have proved it by an experience of nearly four years. It is humane, as all must acknowledge. It contributes to the comfort, the cheerfulness, and the recovery of the insane. It is safe, for no accident has occurred under it with constant *surveillance*. It soothes the patient, keeps his angry and revengeful passions at rest, gives him the power to assist himself, and thereby prevents his falling into habits of hopeless filth and misery ; and I venture to pronounce of it, that it is the system which must and will ultimately prevail in every asylum in our land. I remain, Sir, your obedient and faithful servant,

"ROBERT GARDINER HILL,

" House-Surgeon."

" Lunatic Asylum, Lincoln,
Feb. 14, 1840."

This letter, although merely a defensive reply to the observations in the report of the West Riding of

York Pauper Lunatic Asylum, and containing no personal attack upon any one, drew forth the following observations from Dr Corsellis: (see his letters to the 'Lancet' of March 29th and May 9th, 1840).

"It is true that 'no improvement in science takes place without meeting its opponents.' I add, with all deference, it is equally true that no wild scheme has ever been promulgated, from the days of the miraculously-healing shrines, to the dream of animal magnetism, without finding its supporters; nor has any enthusiast erected his standard, either in the medical or the moral world, without attracting some followers. I copy an extract on the subject of restraint from the Nineteenth Report of the admirably conducted asylum at Dundee, an institution which I recommend to the attention of all who are concerned in the management of the insane.

"In the recent publication of Mr Hill, of the Lincoln Asylum, he asserts, 'that in a properly constructed building, with a sufficient number of suitable attendants, restraint is never necessary, never justifiable, and always injurious in all cases of lunacy whatever.' It is believed that, if this point were to be settled by practical men, Mr Hill would be left in a very small minority. But, even allowing the practicability of the measure, whether it is humane and desirable, is a question which appears to be very problematical.

"We, who have the superintendence of institutions appointed for the treatment of the insane, have a trust confided to us at once the most responsible, painful, and difficult. Our only emulation ought to be, not how we may best exalt ourselves or our system, but how we may most successfully advance the good of the whole; and I am quite sure that, where that real philanthrophy is found which can alone give energy to our efforts, and support us in making them, *there* will be the least arrogant dictation, the most practical good sense, and a becoming professional respect towards those who are labourers with us in the same great cause.

" I should judge Mr Hill, in his praiseworthy zeal, has never tried any system but his own.

" When we shall find those institutions which boast the total abolition of restraint return the largest proportion of cures, and shall have sufficient evidence that the unfortunate inmates are healthier and happier than any others; then, and not until then, will it be time for me, and a host of my respected medical brethren, to acknowledge the system is not a piece of contemptible quackery—a mere bait for the public ear —but really a valuable improvement in science, for which the originators well deserve from the medical profession, and the insane world at large, the warmest thanks and the most profound respect.

(Signed)　　" C. C. CORSELLIS, M.D."

Mr Samuel Hadwen, my predecessor in office at the Lincoln Asylum, was the next to attack my heterodoxy. Of this gentleman, the Rev. W M. Pierce, a Governor of the Lincoln Asylum, asserted in 1851 that, had Mr Hadwen remained at the Asylum a little longer, non-restraint would have been attained without my assistance. His own evidence, however, sufficiently demonstrates the fallacy of this assertion ; for he advocates the use of restraint as a powerful remedial agent in the cure of insanity, and declares that it would be as absurd to attempt to dispense with it, as with medicine in the case of bodily ailments.—See his opinions quoted in Appendix (D).

Mr Pierce endeavoured to detract from the merit of total abolition by representing the reduction of restraints (see his letter to the ' Lancet,' Feb, 1, 1851, and my answer thereto, Feb. 22) to have taken place under Mr Hadwen in the ratio of seven to one. I beg leave to set that matter at rest by introducing the following table, showing the real state of the case.

Year.	Number of Patients under Treatment.	Number of Patients placed under Restraint.	Per centage of Patients restrained.	Per centage of Patients restrained by each House-Surgeon.	Name of House-Surgeon.
1829	72	39	54.16 }		
1830	92	54	58.69 }	56.42½	Mr Thos. Fisher
1831	70	40	57.14 }		
1832	81	55	67.90 }	58.53½	Mr H. Marston
1833	87	44	50.57 }		
1834	109	45	41.28 }		
1835	108	28	25.92 }	32.65	Mr S. Hadwen
1836	115	12	10.43 }		
1837	130	2	1.53 }	7.22	Mr R. G. Hill
1838	158	—	—		

In a letter to the ' Lancet,' in reply to Sir E. F. Bromhead, given in Appendix (C), I published a table showing the result of treatment in the Lincoln Asylum prior to the introduction of non-restraint, viz., from March 16, 1829, to December 1835. That table I will introduce here, because the results are important as bearing upon the question of restraint or non-restraint.

Patients discharged from the Books.	Having been under Restraint.	Not having been under Restraint.	Number of Hours passed under Restraint.	Average Number of Hours under Restraint.	Per centage as effected by		Per centage of Suicides.	Per centage of Deaths from Maniacal Exhaustion.
					Restrnt.	Non-Restrnt.		
Recovered or Improved .... } 161	65	96	23,616	363	40.37	59.62		
Dead 52	44	8	48,394	1,100	84.61	15.38	11.11	9.61
Removed during treatment, escaped, and remaining in Asylum .... } 110	78	32	23,865	306				
Totals 323	187	136	95,875		57.89	42.10		

Of seventeen patients who had been under excessive restraint, I give the following particulars :

Patients' Number.	Sex.	Number of Hours under Restraint.	Period of Treatment.	Termination of Case.
109	Male	5,827	31 months	Death
173	Male	7,542½	31 months	Death
256	Male	4,591½	4½ years	Death
284	Male	4,684¾	5 years	Death
280	Male	1.175	10 months	Death
293	Male	2,691	12 months	Escape
307	Male	2,246	2 years	Death
309	Male	345	12 months	Death
405	Male	198	6 weeks	{ Suicide: burnt himself to death
323	Female	7,985	21 months	Death
394	Female	5,282	17 months	Death
343	Female	1,582	2 months	Suicide: hanged herself
306	Female	1,816½	3 months	Removal by friends
316	Female	2,195½	15 months	Recovery
389	Male	5,730	16 months	Recovery
390	Male	146	7 days	Death
453	Female	956	4 months	Suicide : strangled herself

These cases occurred under a system of mitigation,

and immediately preceding my appointment as House-Surgeon. By the seventeen patients 54,996 hours were passed under restraint, so that each averaged 3,235 hours. The result cannot excite surprise. Deaths, (of which three were by suicide) 13,—escape, 1,—removal by friends, 1,—recoveries, 2,—total, 17. I regret that it is not in my power to give these cases *in extenso ;* I have only the particulars of case 390, and partially so of case 389, which will be found in Appendix (G.)

These particulars show the condition of the Lincoln Asylum under the mitigation system, and very little prior to my connection with it. Mr Pierce, in the controversy which subsequently occurred, affirmed that Dr Charlesworth was the real originator of non-restraint; yet here Dr Charlesworth himself appears as the *inventor* of boot hobbles, for confining the feet to the bottom of the tub bedstead. It has been broadly stated that through the exertions of Dr Charlesworth restraint was merely employed in " exceptional cases ;" that in these cases it was of the mildest kind, and was always removed as early as possible. I have never denied the humane exertions of Dr Charlesworth to mitigate restraint—I always acknowledged them to their full extent:—but when the disingenuous attempt was made to ascribe to Dr Charlesworth the abolition of restraint, or even the intention to abolish it, then I was compelled to refer to the actual state of things in the Lincoln Asylum, even under the " mildest " period of restraint, just prior to my connection with it; and the actual state of the asylum at this juncture proves the truth of Sir E. F. Bromhead's statement, that neither Dr Charlesworth nor any other governor of the asylum ever expected even then the entire abolition of restraint; that they neither asked for it, nor deemed it possible.

Let case 389 (see Appendix G.) speak for itself: — The poor fellow was not only subjected to every species of cruelty, but the restraint was continued for months after he had been brought into a state of *"imbecility,"* *"taking no cognizance of what passed around him,"* *"being led about by the attendant,"* *only able to take* *"moderate exercise,"* and even after the medical super-intendent had reported him as *"not at all violent, and sitting the whole day in a state of childishness."* He is brought into the most abject state of filth and misery, is fastened to a chair, against which he kicks his heels until he has a sore upon one of them, then he gets the handcuff (" the simple method ") twisted so as to make pressure upon his wrist, and a serious injury is the consequence—inflammation follows, and he requires to have eighteen leeches applied, and several poultices; he is chained hands and feet in a tub-bedstead, upon straw, and is unable to assist himself, and lies night after night in his own fœces—the treatment produces sores, and in his attempts to extricate himself his arms become chafed, and then it is found that " the strait-waistcoat is the mildest and most efficient mode of restraint." The patient gets a wound, most probably from a thorn or something sharp amongst the straw, he is covered with sores, and has abscesses of the ear, at the back of his head, and upon other parts of his person. A more loathsome and dreadful spectacle cannot well be imagined, a man in petticoats, for weeks

and months exhibited to his fellow patients, and to the
gaze of strangers led thither, some through curiosity,
others from motives of philanthropy. Taking it for
granted that this was an exceptional case, what neces·
sity was there for restraint, upon the acknowledged
principles of the asylum, *after the patient became
childish?* We will come to the real facts of the case.
The patient is reported in December *as " led about by
an attendant," as "much calmer,"* and *" more manageable,"* and, although in this state, and *with sores upon
almost every part of his person,* and *very weak,* he is
during that month 653 hours under restraint! In
January, when he is said to be *" quite imbecile, taking
no cognizance of what passed around him," requiring to
be led about by the " keeper,"* and reported as *" sitting
the whole day in a state of childishness,"* he is kept
under restraint for 523 hours ! In February, March,
and April, still reported *" childish"* and *" calm,"* he is
in February 308, March 231, and April 330 hours
under restraint, and the following three months 341,
330, and 209 hours respectively! For thirteen months
he underwent every kind of torture, and the number of
hours passed under restraint during that period was
5,730 ! It is really wonderful that he did not share
the fate of the thirteen who were subjected to similar
treatment and died. Subsequently he was free from
any kind of restraint for a period of three months, and
was at length discharged recovered. He returned, however, in a short time, was again under treatment for
four months, and was discharged a second time as recovered. During his last incarceration he was only

once the subject of restraint, and that for about five hours. A short time after his last discharge he was taken ill and died.—And such was the practice of the Lincoln Asylum when I entered upon my duties in 1835.

It will be seen from the report of the Lincoln Asylum for 1835, written in April, about three months preceding my appointment, that the abolition of restraint was not then contemplated : for the report states that " the object of restraint is not punishment, but security." It also states that "the instruments of restraint have been reduced to four mild and simple methods, viz.—

"Day, 1. The wrists secured by a flexible connection, with a belt round the waist.

"2. The ankles secured by a flexible connection with each other, so as to allow of walking exercise.

"Night, 3. One or both wrists attached by a flexible connection to the side of the bed.

"4. The feet placed in night-shoes, similarly attached to the foot of the bed."

Whatever might be said against the use of the strait-waistcoat, it was infinitely preferable to these iron handcuffs and locked chains, for such, in fact, they were, although described, and no doubt intended, as "mild and simple methods " of restraint. I say the old fashioned strait-waistcoat was infinitely preferable to fastenings of this kind at night, because in the one case the patient could get out of bed and attend to the calls of nature, in the other he could not. It was a most filthy and abominable mode of restraint. The bed was what is called a "tub-bed," with boarded sides and ends, and was filled with straw; and in this miserable plight the poor patient (perhaps previously tended with all the care of an anxious and devoted wife), passed the night, unable to assist himself, or even *to change his posture.* The same objection also lies against locking the feet to the foot-board of the bedstead in boots made of ticking, and called " night shoes,"—a mode of restraint invented by Dr Charlesworth, and certainly milder than locking the feet in iron, as the hands were. I have seen, in many instances, the most foul ulcers produced by the constant chafing and struggling against these iron handcuffs.

Then again, by reference to the minutes of the Asylum, it will be seen that, on the 18th of August 1834, the furnishing committee was ordered to take measures for procuring improved wrist-locks for day and night use. That the committee did take the necessary measures I can vouch for them; for within a few months after my appointment I received a large parcel from Birmingham, containing about four dozen steel handcuffs. *These instruments were never used,* and after awhile were sold as " old iron."

The next person who attacked the system, and myself as the author of it, was (singular to say !) Dr William Cookson, one of the physicians of the Asylum, himself at first a supporter of both !—see his letter testimonial to myself, Appendix (B.) The attack was exceedingly violent and personal, and was carried on for a long period. It was during this attack that I withdrew from the superintendence of the Asylum, where insubordination, thus encouraged, was the order of the day, and all control at an end. I had no access to the Board-room, andconsequently could not defend myself or the system. I therefere withdrew from the management, qualified as a governor, and entered the arena with Dr Cookson on equal terms. The fight was hot and fierce. Ultimately Dr Cookson confessed himself mistaken. His recantation of his accusations against the system, made about a month prior to his decease, and entered by himself on the minutes of the Asylum, was a manly act, and does immortal honour to his memory !*

The system at this time encountered a furious storm of opposition, new opponents sprang up almost daily :— their name was Legion. Dr Clutterbuck denounced it as " empirical, and highly dangerous to the patient and to those around him." Dr James Johnson believed that, " if the magistrates who advocated the non-restraint system were to see a patient in a furor, they would change their opinion; the system in question indicated insanity on the part of its supporters; it was *a mania*, which,

---

* Dr Cookson *On Non-Restraint.*—" One declaration I feel it but candid and manly to make before I close this book for ever. An observation of many months has convinced me that the defects I formerly thought inherent, necessarily inherent, on the non-restraint system, and inseparable from it, are not so, and, with few exceptions, may be considered referrible to other and to extraneous sources. I do not mean to fly from one extreme to another, and to say that the system is perfect. I am convinced that much is to be discovered, and much will be discovered, but in a moment like this, which, to me, is not without its solemnity, I should consider the suppression of any change of opinion on a subject like this a sacrifice to self, and consequently unworthy. (Signed) " W. D. Cookson."

like others, would have its day." Sir Alexander
Morison, one of the physicians of Bethlem Hospital, and
visiting physician of the Surrey County Lunatic Asylum,
said "it was a gross and palpable absurdity, the wild
scheme of a philanthropic visionary, unscientific and
impossible."* It was denounced, too, by Dr Blake and
Mr Powell, of the Nottingham Asylum; by Dr Millingen,
late Medical Superintendent of the Middlesex County
Asylum at Hanwell; by Dr Stewart, of the Belfast
Asylum; Dr McKintosh, of Dundee; Dr Browne, of
Dumfries; and a host of minor opponents. To reply to
all their various objections was impossible; but it is a
singular fact that some of those who objected to the
system most strongly were amongst its earliest converts!
I may make honourable mention, e. g., of the superin-

---

* Happily for mankind, the state of Bethlem at that time is now
(thanks to the wild scheme of a philanthropic visionary), "impossible"! It was then a disgrace to the nation! and yet when, in consequence of the disclosures made through the investigations carried on,
the visiting physicians were discharged, and Dr Hood was appointed
resident physician, Sir Alexander Morison received a pension of 150l.
per annum, a sum greater than is given in many instances, I grieve to
say, to the resident superintendents of our large public asylums!
Under such circumstances one would have supposed that an honourable
mind would have shrunk from receiving a pension at all! Since the
appointment of Dr Hood great improvements have been going on at
Bethlem; even the "gross and palpable absurdity" of non-restraint
has found its way thither. Why was Sir A. Morison, after having
been discharged from Bethlem, retained as visiting physician at the
Surrey County Asylum? Visiting physicians are in most instances
useless appendages, for the responsibility must necessarily rest with
the resident-superintendent. The office of visiting physician, if retained,
should be an honorary appointment, under the Commissioners in
Lunacy; and might thus, perhaps, be some check upon any mismanage-
ment of the institution.

tendents of the Dundee and Glasgow Asylums. I am not sure whether Dr Stewart subsequently became a convert to the non-restraint system. Dr Corsellis, I am aware, never changed his opinion, but adhered to the old system to the very last. It was curious, however, to see his name in the list of subscribers to the Conolly Testimonial. The Wakefield Asylum has now the advantage of being conducted by Mr Alderson, under the very system which elicited so much hostility on the part of his predecessor.

The following extracts contain the views of Dr Blake, the late Mr Powell, Dr Millingen, and Dr Stewart.

From the Thirtieth Report of the General Lunatic Asylum, Nottingham, 1840.—" It has been our anxious wish, in the course of our treatment, to use the least possible personal restraint; for although we continue to regard ' the total abolition of all restraint' in the cure of insanity as altogether an ' utopian proposal,' yet our experience has long ago led us to the conclusion that the necessity for its application is comparatively very rare.

(Signed) " ANDREW BLAKE, M.D.
" THOMAS POWELL."

From Dr Andrew Blake's Letter to the ' Lancet,' Dec. 19, 1840.—" Mr Hill, the late Director of the Lincoln Lunatic Asylum, was the first to broach the *total abolition* doctrine in this country, and, as such, he deserves some credit, inasmuch as, although it may not be found practicable to the full extent of its meaning, yet, by rousing the attention of persons in charge of lunatics to the consideration of the subject, much good has and will be the result. This gentleman, in his little work, headed 'total abolition of personal restraint in the treatment of the insane,' says, at page 21, 'I wish to complete that which Pinel began; I assert, then, in plain and distinct terms, *that in a properly constructed building*, with a sufficient number of suitable attendants, restraint is never necessary, never justifiable, and *always injurious* in all cases of *lunacy whatsoever.*' Mr Hill has, by this declaration, as it were, nailed his colours to the mast-head, and staked his reputation on its truth. * * * * In the twenty-ninth report of the Nottingham General Lunatic Asylum, the director of that institution and I stated our opinions on this subject in the following terms:—' We cannot, however, conclude without alluding to what we expressed in our reports of last year, with regard to the utopian proposal of the *total abolition of all restraint* in the treatment of insanity, as has been advocated in a recent publication. We do so, because we are still of opinion that it is, like all other extremes, neither judicious nor practicable; our experience, on the contrary, while it teaches us to condemn *all unnecessary restraint*, has led us to consider its *well-timed application*, as being not unfrequently peculiarly useful as a powerful agent in the moral treatment of insanity; and further, we assert that cases do occur in which it is impossible to dispense with it without exposing the patient to imminent danger.'

(Signed)   " ANDREW BLAKE, M.D."

From Dr Millingen's ' Aphorisms on the Treatment and Management of the Insane,' p. 106, 1840.—" Except in cases of violent mania, restraint is rarely necessary; unless it be to prevent the mischievous idiot and the maniac from destroying property, when gentle restraint is required to prevent them from constantly tearing their clothes and bedding, or breaking the window panes, or anything they can lay hold of. *It may, however, be occasionally employed as a punishment, the dread of which keeps many lunatics in order.*

" Nothing can be more absurd, speculative, or peculative, than the attempts of theoretic visionaries, or candidates for popular praise, to do away with all restraint. Desirable as such a management might be, it can never prevail without much danger to personal security, and a useless waste and dilapidation of property."

From Dr Robert Stewart's Letter to the ' Lancet,' May 1, 1841.—" I am not a disciple of the total abolition school, my deliberate opinion on this head being that instrumental restraint,—by which I by no means intend ' iron hobbles, chains, beatings or bruisings,' such as Mr Hill, of Lincoln, averred to be the species of restraint in common use in English lunatic asylums— cannot, either with safety or humanity, be dispensed with altogether ; but, on the contrary, that its occasional and judicious application is not only unavoidable in many instances, but is a most valuable curative means, if confided to humane and professionally educated superintendents who, considering the great and unceasing responsibility of their arduous office, ought assuredly to be permitted free agency as to its use or disuse, equally so as in the prescribing of the most fitting *medical treatment* for such unhappy, but very perplexing, cases as require restraint being had recourse to. Surely it will not be denied that such distinguished and ex-perienced men in the management of the insane as Dr Corsellis (Wakefield), Dr Kirkman (Suffolk), Dr Blake and Surgeon Powell (Nottingham), Drs Browne, Hutchinson, McKinnon, Malcolm, &c. &c., of the Scotch Asylums, should not be entrusted with this free agency? And is their humanity to be called into ques-tion by anonymous writers, forsooth, because, in the exercise of a sound discretion, they summon restraint to their aid? Away with such mock tenderness, such morbid sympathy, and sensitiveness for the furious insane; through evil report and good report, I trust the above individuals will continue to pursue the even tenor of their way, and by so doing be preserved from the dangerous hallucinations of that monomania of the present day, non-restraintism, which, of all others, calls loudly for prompt and close restraint, so as to keep its unfortunate patients within the bounds of moderation.

(Signed) "ROBERT STEWART, M.D.,
"Medical Superintendent of the Belfast
District Lunatic Asylum."

From Mr Powell's Letter to the 'Lancet,' April, 24, 1841.—"From the perusal of this paragraph, any reader would conclude that. Dr Stewart was a decided and unflinching supporter of the new doctrine for the

D

management of asylums ; what the doctor's real opinions
are, I leave you and your readers to judge from the
tenor of two letters which I have been favoured with,
and which I transcribe, having obtained the authors'
permission to do so.

" 'Belfast Asylum, Jan. 13, 1841.—Dear Sir,—I
shall feel greatly obliged by your letting me have a
copy of your late (30th) report of the General Asylum
at Nottingham for the reception of Lunatics, some
extracts from which I have lately read in the ' Lancet,'
and have been very happy to find that you and your
colleague, Dr Blake, do not advocate that most preposterous proposition of the present day, that restraint
is injurious and unnecessary in every case of lunacy
whatever ! !

"ROBERT STEWART, M.D.' "

" 'Belfast Asylum, March 31, 1841.—My Dear
Sir,—I have this day received your kind favour of the
28th, and lose no time in replying to it. I have not
yet been supplied with the ' Lancet' of the 27th inst.,
consequently have not read the letter signed " a Medical
Superintendent," in which my humble name has been
introduced by the writer's quotation of a paragraph
from my report of this asylum for last year relative to
the restraint question, and although *prima facie* the
quotation brought forward, and that portion of my
communication addressed to yourself privately (which
you have kindly quoted for me), may appear inconsistent, if not contradictory ; yet, on the other hand, when
such is fairly compared, it strikes me that nothing of

the kind can be laid to my charge, as it must be plainly seen that in stating " that the sooner the restraint system was superseded by the total abolition plan the better, &c. &c.;" I was merely going on the belief that "grievous cruelties" were constantly in operation in the English Asylums from Mr Hill's affirmations and faithful picture of "iron hobbles" (query, what are they?) "beatings, bruisings, and chainings in bed; " and therefore had no hesitation in giving it as my opinion that, fraught as the non-restraint plan was with danger, it would be better to adopt it than to permit such monstrous, faithful pictures to continue in operation.

" 'Having, then, thus explained myself to you, I can have no objection whatever to your quoting the words you have referred to in your intended notice of the letter of " a Medical Superintendent"; I make it my business to read attentively all that appears on this *quæstio vexata* in the 'Lancet,' your colleague Dr Blake's letters amongst the rest, but I am still as far away as ever from being a convert to the Hill-ite doctrine, that restraint is never necessary, &c. &c.

" ROBERT STEWART, M.D.' "

" These opinions, privately communicated to me, lose none of their force when placed in juxta-position with extracts from the report itself; in the ninth page of it, Dr Stewart, after noticing the Middlesex and Lincoln Asylums as being those in which it is stated that the ' total abolition system' has been adopted with the best effects, and comparing these statements with the opinions of Dr Corsellis of the Wakefield Asylum, and Dr Browne of the Dundee, sums up by saying—'Such, then, are the deliberate and publicly-recorded opinions of the heads of two establishments many years in operation, and of well-deserved celebrity, as to the inutility, and, in short, inhumanity, of the total abolition of restraint, *opinions in which the manager of this asylum fully agrees, both as to their entire soundness as well as to their true humanity and wisdom, and cannot express his own views on the point at issue better than by adopting them as his own, and that to the letter.*' In the tenth page of the same report we find a history of two cases, the one of suicidal, the other of homicidal mania, of a most fearful character; and after reciting their peculiar symptoms, we find the same Dr Stewart expressing himself thus:—' In a case like this, and when under the dominion of such paroxysms, would moral influence, it is asked seriously, have any effect? It is *utopian*, in the highest degree, to think so; and to endeavour to practise it would be nothing short of courting the risk of being morally, if not legally, guilty of a breach of the sixth commandment, on the part of any superintendent of an asylum who would thus recklessly dare to peril the lives committed to his charge, by carrying into effect so sweepingly wild an assertion, as that 'restraint is never necessary, never justifiable, and always injurious in all cases of insanity whatever.'

(Signed)   "Thomas Powell,

" Medical Superintendent of the Nottingham Lunatic Asylum."

It may not be amiss here calmly to inquire what there was in the proposal to abolish restraint that could reasonably be expected to draw down upon its author such a mass of bitter invective and personal abuse? It was perhaps natural that the attendants should not be favourable to it, for it entailed an increased amount of vigilant care and labour upon them both by day and night: but for this reason I advocated a proportionate increase in the number and a more liberal remuneration of those attendants. The only answer I can imagine possible to the question is, that when the practicability was demonstrated of treating large numbers of lunatics without any restraint whatever, it seemed to imply some indirect censure upon those who continued to use it. But if this feeling existed, why did they not also discard restraint, instead of railing against those who did? And instead of arguing against the possibility of what had been proved possible by others, why did they not give the new system a fair trial? I believe, where such a trial has been made, the attempt in no one instance has proved abortive.

With the demonstrated success and general adoption of the non-restraint system, the storm of opposition ceased of course; but only to take a new and un-expected direction.

II. In the year 1850, the non-restraint system having been then triumphantly established as the system of all our greatest and best conducted asylums, and Dr Charlesworth having declared at the annual meeting of the Provincial Medical and Surgical Society, that " the real honour of introducing the system belonged to Mr Hill," it was proposed to give a public testimonial to myself as its author; "in connection with which it would seem desirable," the Committee stated, "that the attention of the public be called to this mode of treatment, as worthy of national adoption."

The circulars in which this announcement was made could not, one would have supposed, have given umbrage to any individual. But the proposal itself elicited an amount of angry and jealous feeling which could not possibly have been anticipated, and which has not yet, I fear, entirely subsided. As long as the entire abolition of restraint was considered by some as a doubtful experiment, and by others stigmatized under every possible form of abuse and misrepresentation, no governor of the asylum challenged the claim which they themselves, indeed, had been the first to announce to the public in their reports, and which their own signatures had repeatedly attested. Yet, strange to say! no sooner had this proposal been issued, than the Rev. W. M. Pierce, whose signature as chairman was attached to the first public announcement of my sentiments on the practicability of an entire abolition of restraint, wrote a letter to the editor of the 'Lancet,' wherein he asserted that "the true author and originator of non-restraint" was that very "Dr Charlesworth," who had just declared at Hull, that "the real honour of first introducing the system belonged to Mr Hill!" This letter, together with the controversy to which it led, and the part which Dr Charlesworth took in that controversy, is given in Appendix (D.)

On the publication of the proceedings at the meeting of the Provincial Medical and Surgical Association at Hull, I felt bound, in gratitude, to notice the honourable testimony of Dr Charlesworth in my favour. Accordingly I addressed a letter to the ' Lancet,' which concluded thus :—

" But my especial object in writing to you at present is thus publicly to thank Dr Charlesworth for his honourable avowal, at the late dinner of the Provincial Medical and Surgical Association at Hull,· of the justness of my claims ; and also Dr John Conolly, for his kind and handsome mention of my services. It cannot fail to be gratifying to myself to have *their* public testimony to the fact, that I originated the system which Dr Conolly and others have since carried out upon so large a scale and with such beneficial results—results which will ensure the permanent continuance of the system of non-restraint when its author shall be forgotten in the chambers of the grave "

This, to my infinite astonishment, drew forth a reply from Sir Ed. Ff. Bromhead, above all persons in the world, in which he ventures to state that " no individual could exclusively claim the merit " of abolishing instrumental restraint ! Yet in the same letter he avows,—what he had in other and still stronger terms, if possible, always before avowed,— that " it was Mr Hill, who had the courage to broach the original and invaluable idea, that ' the use of instruments might be WHOLLY dispensed with ! ! ' "

An examination of the documents produced in

Appendices (C.) and (D.), will convince every impartial and unprejudiced mind,* that the opposition
*now first made, after a period of thirteen or fourteen
years,* to my just claims, had its origin in unworthy
motives, and will add no lustre to the names of Sir
E. Ff. Bromhead, the Rev. W. M. Pierce, nor (I
regret to be obliged to add) of Dr Charlesworth
himself.

In reference to this attempt, which excited the
just indignation of all who were conversant with the
facts of the case, the Rev. J. Daniel, one of the
Secretaries to the Testimonial Committee, thus expresses himself in a letter to the Editor of the
' Medical Gazette,' dated October 14th, 1851 :

" The simple unbiassed history of the abolition of
restraint is contained in the Reports of the Lincoln
Asylum for the years 1837 and 1838, drawn up by
Dr Charlesworth, and signed respectively by Mr
Pierce and himself, as the Chairmen. It was not,
therefore, an uninformed or misguided set of directors,
who gave Mr Hill the credit of originating " non-
restraint," but it was assigned to him by that very
physician upon whom Mr Pierce would *now, in direct
contradiction to his own testimony in* 1837, most
willingly ' *thrust the honour.*' WHY ? *Because the
system has triumphed over all opposition ;* and, by
the force of its intrinsic worth, has established itself
throughout the length and breadth of the land. Had
it *failed,* no Mr Pierce would have claimed it for

* See the letter of Dr H. Van Leeuwen, an entire stranger to
myself, inserted in Appendix (E.)

Dr Charlesworth :—the signature of 1837, ' W. M. Pierce, Chairman,' would have proved the ' rash' attempt to be the 'raving of the theoretic visionary' Mr Hill ; and the ' cautious and philosophic Dr Charlesworth' would have had the credit of having given the ' Utopian ' system a fair trial."

The conduct of Dr Charlesworth was utterly in-explicable. He not only declined to be on the Committee, but in the face of all evidence, of the reports of every journal that recorded the speech,— the 'Provincial Medical and Surgical Journal,' the organ of the society,—the 'Lancet,' the local and county papers, the evidence of Drs Robertson, Munro, Heygate,* &c., " ratified," as Dr Robertson remarks, " by the unanimous assent and approval of that numerous meeting,"—in the face of all this evidence, he declared that he " doubted" whether he had expressed himself in those exact terms or not ! although they expressed no more than what he had over and over again stated before !—This con-duct excited a strong feeling of indignation, and was publicly and deservedly reprobated.

For myself, I could scarcely believe it possible ; but " to make assurance doubly sure," I addressed the following letter to Dr Charlesworth, who certainly had not of late shown me the same kind attention which had been invariably his practice hitherto.

* See the letters of these gentlemen inserted in Appendices (B.) and (D.)

" To E. P. Charlesworth, Esq., Senior Physician to the Lincoln Lunatic Asylum :—

" Dear Sir,—An attack having been made by your friend Mr Pierce upon my claim to be the originator of the total abolition of instrumental restraint in the Lincoln Lunatic Asylum, in the ' Lancet ' of Feb. 1st ; and that attack having been repeated in the ' Lancet ' of March 1st ; and now again by means of Sir A. Morison's letter, inserted by Mr Pierce in the ' Stamford Mercury ' of the 11th of April, I feel compelled to ask you if these attacks were made with your knowledge, and with your approbation.—I am, dear Sir, yours faithfully,   " ROBERT GARDINER HILL.

" Eastgate House, April 17th, 1851."

To which I received the same day the following reply :—

" Sir,—I beg to acknowledge your communication of this date, and am, Sir, your obedient servant,
                    " E. P. CHARLESWORTH.

" Lincoln, April 17th, 1851.

" To R. G. Hill, Esq."

Will it be believed that this is the same Dr Charlesworth who, a short time prior to the proposed testimonial, had " frankly avowed himself " to Dr Granville, " the *staunchest advocate* of the plan" of non-restraint, " as well as of the *originator* of it !"
—(See Dr Granville's Spas of England, Midland Division, p. 87.)

In October, 1851, the controversy having re-
sulted in the triumphant vindication of the truth,
the presentation of the proposed testimonial took
place at Lincoln. It consisted of a very handsome
silver centre-piece, with a circular plinth, ornamented
with festoons ; around the base are three elegant
female figures, in frosted silver, supporting a basket
for flowers. Upon one of the panels is engraved
the following :

> " Presented, together with a silver tea-service, to
> Robert Gardiner Hill, Esq., M.R.C.S. Eng.,
> author and originator of the total abolition
> of restraint in the treatment of the insane,
> now commonly called the 'Non-restraint
> system,' by a number of subscribers, medical
> and general, from all parts of the kingdom,
> in token of their admiration of the talent
> which could devise, and the energy and
> patient perseverance which, despite of pre-
> judice, opposition, and jealousy, could carry
> out a system fraught with results so eminently
> beneficial to mankind."

On the opposite side are inscribed the following
extracts :—

> " The Governors never expressed a wish for the
> extinction of restraints ; they never expected
> it ; not one of them deemed it possible. "
> " It was 'Mr Hill who had the courage to broach
> the original and invaluable idea, that the
> use of instruments might be wholly dis-

pensed with.'—Sir E. Ff Bromhead, Bart.,
Vice-President of the Lincoln Asylum."

"The real honour belonged to Mr Hill, of the
Lincoln Asylum.—Dr Charlesworth."

I crave permission here to insert my reply, because
it bears upon many of the points mooted in the late
controversy.

"Mr Chairman, Ladies, and Gentlemen,—In accepting this superb token of your approval, I feel that
I cannot express one half of what my heart would
dictate. I have, it is true, laboured hard, and suffered
much, but this expression of your appreciation of those
labours is an abundant reward. For I regard not
merely the worth and value of this elegant and costly
present, but what is to me a much greater consideration
than even this, I regard it as a token and pledge that
you consider that system of treating insanity which I
had the happiness of discovering, as a boon to a large
and unfortunate class of sufferers, and as a step in the
onward progress of humanity.

"You have a fair right to inquire by what process
I arrived at the important conclusion which I announced
many years ago in my published Lecture on the total
abolition of restraint in the treatment of the insane:—
viz. ' That in a properly constructed building, with a
sufficient number of suitable attendants, restraint is
never necessary, never justifiable, and always injurious,
in all cases of lunacy whatever.' I will endeavour to
explain some of the steps by which I was led to adopt
this theory, which I announced in such general and
confident terms.

" It is scarcely necessary for me to remind you, because I have frequently stated the fact, that at the period I was appointed House-Surgeon to the Lincoln Lunatic Asylum, and for some years previously, the system of treatment constantly urged upon the attention of the Boards by the humane and talented physician of the establishment, Dr Charlesworth, was that of a *mitigation* of restraint as far as was deemed consistent with safety. But still *the system was one of restraint;* nay more, restraint was *an essential element* in it, for even in April, 1835, only about three months previously to my appointment, restraint was declared to be *essential to safety.* ' The object of restraint is not punishment, but security,' observes the report of that year. ' The Governors,' says Sir Edward Ff. Bromhead, ' did what they could in a proper direction: *they mitigated evil.'* In these words, Sir Edward Ffrench Bromhead accurately describes the system of the Lincoln Lunatic Asylum previously to my appointment. ' *They mitigated evil;*' but the total abolition of restraint was not contemplated. Safety, without restraint, in all cases was not deemed possible; and, if I may be allowed to say so, the great merit of my discovery consists in my having demonstrated, that not only was safety consistent with ' non-restraint,' but that *the only safe system* was that of *non-restraint*—that, in truth, *with regard to the patients,* ' a maximum of restraint was *safer than a medium,* and a minimum of restraint *safer than either.'* I say, that in this consists the great merit of the discovery, because the safety of non-restraint being demonstrated, even common sense will point out that innumerable cases of lunacy have some chance of recovery under non-restraint, which must sink into idiotcy, or hopeless imbecility, *under restraint:* the patient being in many cases rendered incapable of self-control, or even of attending to his natural wants.

"Another preliminary remark I have to make is, that the term 'non-restraint' has been used by some of my opponents in a sense which is utterly repugnant to the meaning of the term itself,—that is, to express a *mitigation of restraint.* The word, as applied to the treatment of lunacy, was coined by myself, to express the total abolition of all instrumental restraint, and all severity towards the patients, and was always used by me in this sense alone. I called my plan 'the no-restraint theory,'—a term which explains itself, but which was afterwards expressed by the more euphonious but *strictly synonymous* term 'non-restraint.' This observation is a sufficient answer to the accusation so unjustly made against me, that I wish to 'absorb all the credit' of *amelioration* as well as *total abolition* in my own person. Indeed the most painful, as well as unforeseen circumstance connected with the present valued testimonial is, that the very friends who have in the strongest terms acknowledged the justice of my claims—nay, who themselves, at the time when I made the discovery, cheerfully accorded me the merit of the authorship of the system, without the necessity of any claim on my part, have on the present occasion, from an unworthy feeling of envy, either withheld their coun-tenance or determinedly opposed me. My support and consolation is, that neither they nor any one else can disprove one iota of the evidence upon which my right to the organisation of non-restraint rests : they cannot impugn the irrefragable testimony which renders the truth so clear that it cannot, to investigating minds, be rendered mystical and dubious by the ingenuities of clever sophists—they cannot erase from the journals of the asylum the simple narrative there recorded of the introduction of non-restraint by me, *at the time it was introduced*, and to which their own signatures are affixed. Nor can they bring forward *one single document* in proof of the assertion which *one* individual, and *one alone*, has had the boldness to make, in the very face of his own recorded testimony and of the public disclaimer of Dr Charlesworth, that that gentleman is the originator of non-restraint. You, my friends,— and I think I may add the public generally, and all at least who have taken the trouble to examine the evidence, are convinced of these facts ; but in the midst of the gratification which your kindness gives me, I could not forbear thus far alluding to the very unhandsome way in which I have lately been treated. But of this no more.

" The first thing that struck me on my introduction to the Asylum was a poor fellow with poultices on his wrists, and an attendant standing by him to prevent his eating them. The wrists were poulticed in consequence of injuries produced by the use of handcuffs ; an abscess had formed, and the parts were bruised and excoriated. This patient was imbecile, and harmless, though somewhat inclined to mischief, which was the

reason for his being restrained. This case made a deep
impression upon me, inexperienced as I then was. This
impression was heightened by observing the frequent
struggles and violent efforts made by patients to resist
the imposition of instruments of restraint,—their sufferings under it,—the injuries they inflicted on themselves,— and the spirit of revenge and gloomy resentment
which they nourished against the attendants. It is true,
Dr Charlesworth attempted to improve the instruments
of restraint, by substituting iron handcuffs, and leathern
hobbles for the strait-waistcoat, &c. But after all, it is
doubtful whether this was any very great improvement
upon the old system. I can speak from experience. I
have seen as much mischief result from them as could
possibly have arisen from the use of the strait-waistcoat.
Dr Charlesworth, and Sir Edward Ffrench Bromhead
(in particular), well know that I did not broach the
theory of wholly dispensing with restraint, until I had
literally lived amongst the patients, until I had watched
them by day and by night, and witnessed the dire
effects of even the 'four simple methods of restraint.'
Yes, I have witnessed the torture, the horrifying and
deadly effects of the use of the iron handcuffs and
leg·locks (the means placed at my disposal, and
described in the Report of 1835, as 'simple methods'):
—I have seen the poor maniac under the gripe of the
instruments, writhing, straining, and struggling to get
free :—I have seen the agonising sweat, the distorted
eyes, the veins of the head and neck swollen, the
arms and ankles inflamed, bruised and excoriated:
—I have seen the utter helplessness to which the

patient has been reduced, followed by bed-sores, exhaustion, and death. Never shall I forget the sufferings of A. B. A period of two or three months had elapsed without the use of any coercion whatever, when in an unguarded moment I gave way to the solicitations of the attendants, and this poor creature was handcuffed and hobbled, and placed in solitary confinement; there he remained for some days, howling, yelling, shouting, and blaspheming, until at last he broke out of his cell, shivering the door to pieces. He was then chained to his bedstead, according to the 'simple methods' recommended in April 1835. In this case, I witnessed all these results of treatment, until at last he sunk, a prey to the fatal system. This case determined me as to my future proceedings: no male patient, *i. e.* no patient on the completed side of the house, was ever after put under restraint, except one for about eight hours in my absence. I felt certain, and I do so still, that had this poor fellow been differently treated, he might have been still alive, and in all probability restored to his family. Reflecting on these things, and finding that good effects invariably followed a milder treatment, I made statistical tables with great labour; I tabulated the results of different modes of treatment ; I considered the several cases individually ; I lived amongst the patients ; I watched their habits ; I reflected that sometimes for days together restraint had been dispensed with, although the principle had not been adopted, nor thought of, as applied to the more violent cases. At length, I announced my confident belief that under a proper system of surveillance, with

E

a suitable buiding, instrumental restraint was in every case unnecessary and injurious. I mentioned this opinion to Dr Charlesworth and the Governors; I adopted it as a principle; I acted upon it; and I verified my theory by carrying it into effect.

"But now arose a perfect hurricane of opposition to myself and my system, within the institution and without. I was abused in no measured terms; and the Hill-ite system denominated ' speculative, ' ' peculative,' ' Utopian,' &c. &c., ' the raving of a theoretic visionary,' and, by unnecessarily exposing the lives of the attendants, a practical breaking of the 6th commandment. Nevertheless, the system was carried on *with safety*, and with results which cannot be too highly appreciated. Not a single instance of suicide has occurred in the asylum since the adoption of this system, although they were not infrequent under the mitigation system; proving that, as regards the patients themselves, even a maximum of restraint was safer than a medium; and that nothing but constant surveillance by day and by night can prevent suicide under any system whatever. Moreover, insensible patients required habits of self-control, which is one great step towards cure; the proportion of recoveries increased, comfort and good order prevailed in the place of noise and uproar, and not one fatal accident occurred. Every subsequent year, and every fresh trial, has demonstrated the value and safety of the system. It has triumphed by its own intrinsic worth against prejudice, opposition, and calumny of every kind; and although the violence of the opposition within the institution, in which 'non-restraint' originated, at length compelled me to resign my situation; and although I was shut out from some other important posts because I was the author of that 'absurd dogma' that *restraint is never necessary*, yet I have lived to see that 'absurd dogma' established as the principle of almost every large and well-conducted asylum in the kingdom." (See 'Stamford and Rutland Mercury,' Nov. 7, 1851.)

And here I might close this short sketch, but I cannot help availing myself of an opportunity which may not recur of making a few observations connected with the subject, or bearing upon the improved mode of treating the insane, and

1st. It is the existence of these controversies in different publications, and in detached parts, and a knowledge of the effects which they have had, where they are thus imperfectly known, which have determined me to republish the lecture I delivered in 1839, together with this introductory sketch, and appendices containing documentary evidence, and a full account of the great controversy which arose out of the proposal to present this testimonial. That this controversy had its origin in a spirit of jealousy utterly unworthy of such an occasion, is too lamentably evident. And never, I should imagine, did any controversy arise under similar circumstances, where the opponents were thoroughly aware of the facts of the case, and were convicted by their own previous *unbiassed* testimony *freely and voluntarily given at the time!*

2ndly. Although the controversies referred to put me to an enormous expense in vindicating my claims against the unjust and inconsistent attacks of Sir Edward Ffrench Bromhead, Mr Pierce, and others, and although I regretted exceedingly at the time that my name should have been so frequently dragged before the public, yet, I had the consolation of knowing that this occurred through no fault of mine, as I have before explained; and I had the further consolation of reflecting that, harassed and worried to death as I was, a great and permanent good had been effected; and this was something.*   A mighty reform was brought about

---

* It is a most remarkable fact that within a few years after I had ceased to be connected with the Lincoln Asylum, a retrograde movement commenced there, in the very birth-place of non-restraint. Classification, so necessary towards good management, and to the successful working of the non-restraint system, and so strongly insisted upon by Dr Charlesworth in the earlier periods of the asylum, was at his instigation broken up some six or seven years prior to his decease; and since then all have associated together, the quiet and inoffensive and the convalescent being compelled to mix with the violent and the more troublesome patients. The reports of the Lincoln Asylum for 1846 and 1847 advocate the disuse of classification; the result however was anything but advantageous to the patients, and tended, with other changes, to lower the high repute in which the asylum had previously stood, since the introduction of non-restraint. (See the leading article in the 'Times,' Oct. 15th, 1847; Also Dr Tuke's Prize Essay on the 'Moral Management of the Insane,' p. 85.) About the same time an attempt was made to resist the visitation of the Commissioners in Lunacy.   And now a word with reference to asylums under the management of a Committee of gentlemen, as *e. g.* the Lincoln Asylum. God forbid that they should become general—good management for a continuance is quite out of the question in such institutions. There is too much rivalry, too much jealousy, too much favouritism, and constant bickerings. If a vacancy occurs in the office of Superintendent, the patients may be sacrificed for the purpose of serving a friend. This

in the treatment of the insane, which, I am bold to say, must be still further developed:—*Non-restraint must be madecompulsory:*—*Instruments of torture must no longer be found in any asylum, either public or private.* With regard to private asylums, it is urged that restraint cannot be abolished in the whole of these establishments, on account of the limited size of some of them. No asylum should contain mixed classes. It should be either for the upper, the middle, or the lower classes. If for the upper, the payments will afford the means, the size of the building being quite out of the question. If for the middle, the building should accommodate from eighty to one hundred patients, since no proprietor with ten, twenty, or thirty patients of this class could afford the requisite attendance, as

---

was the case at Lincoln, a circumstance that will partly account for the retrograde movement there. A very worthless fellow was elected to the office of Superintendent, because he was the friend of the Rev. Mr Pierce. Under this superintendent, in 1846, the greatest enormities were practised; enormities that would scarcely be thought possible in the present day. The asylum for many months was the constant scene of obscenities, drunkenness and riot; and this was going on under the eyes of some three or four acting governors, the officers, and servants; and no steps were taken to put a stop to it. At length the gentleman's conduct became the general subject of conversation in the City, and he was at last told that, if he did not resign, he would be dismissed, and he resigned accordingly. Will it be believed that *this man was afterwards received as a visitor at the asylum!* During his visit he managed to steal a gold watch belonging to a patient, and for this offence he was tried and sentenced to three months' imprisonment. With such irregularities it cannot be matter of surprise, that the asylum has sunk in public estimation. Any other person would have been summarily dismissed. One thing is clear, that such a state of things would not be tolerated in a private asylum, for the Commissioners would at once withdraw the licence.

the payments seldom exceed a guinea a week. No licence should be granted unless it can be shown that, either from the size of the building, or the payments, or both combined, the patients may receive the comforts, care, and attention to which they are entitled, and which humanity will accord to them. It will be seen, on reference to the accounts of pauper asylums, that the larger the number of patients, the smaller is the weekly charge. If therefore the above suggestion, founded on the same principle, were complied with in the case of private asylums, it would enable the proprietor to be more liberal, to increase the number of his attendants, and thus to give every patient the free and unshackled use of his limbs, in a manner perfectly consistent with safety, and conducive, more than any other thing, to his speedy restoration. In establishments with small means, mechanical contrivances are mere substitutes for vigilance; the latter is attended with expense, the former can be had at a trifling cost. The only effectual remedy against this evil would be the removal of all patients thus treated to houses conducted without restraint. The Commissioners have already done much good in this way as far as their powers extend ; and if this plan were generally adopted, we should soon cease to hear of the necessity for restraint even in the smallest private asylums.

That instances of mal-treatment still linger, I have lately had ocular proof, in two cases removed from asylums where there was no resident medical officer. Without entering into particulars, I would only observe, that nothing could more strongly demonstrate the necessity of such residence. Ladies, generally speaking, do not possess the combination of qualities necessary for such a position. They cannot be expected to have the tact, the firmness, the determination, presence of mind, and courage, requisite for the management of lunatics; and the result is—the patients suffer—restraint is the expedient resorted to. As, however, no general rule is without an exception, so neither is this. A few ladies there are of extraordinary strength and vigour of mind, capable of grappling with any difficulty: such was Mrs Bowden, late of the Hanwell Asylum, who in the early days of non-restraint achieved wonders in her department of that large institution.

Two things have operated injuriously, and indeed I may fairly say, degraded this part of medical practice: First, the fact that *paupers* have been taken with a view to profit; and Secondly, that non-professional men have speculated in private asylums.

No licence ought to be granted to any non-professional person on any pretext whatever; nor to ladies, except perhaps the widows of professional men who have been engaged in this department of science; and then only with the express understanding that a properly-qualified medical officer should *reside* on the premises, whose orders with regard to medicine, diet, and general management should be imperative.

3. I am very anxious to see the Commissioners in Lunacy invested with more authority. In the granting of licences, why should their powers be limited to London and the neighbourhood? Why not extend them to the whole Kingdom? Provincial houses should be

placed on the same footing as the Metropolitan ; and parties receiving only one patient should be visited ; but for these purposes it would be necessary to enlarge the commission. Great and beneficial results would accrue from the adoption of this plan; for local magistrates cannot be expected to act upon the same views and principles as the Commissioners in Lunacy would. Laymen should not be allowed to take single patients, and medical men receiving such patients into their houses should be licensed. If fifteen pounds be the sum for licensing a house receiving two patients, let the person who receives one patient pay 7*l.* 10s. The single patient requires just as much protection as the others. It is quite shocking to see the condition in which some of these poor creatures are brought to our asylums, sometimes with large sloughs upon their backs, insensible to the calls of nature, and almost in a moribund state. In the present day any discharged attendant thinks himself entitled to a single patient, and the consequence is, that such patients are subjected to all sorts of privations; they have neither recreation, nor amusement, nor exercise, nor have they the free use of their limbs; and the majority are shut up in garrets, tortured with the heat of those apartments in summer, and nearly starved to death in winter, and perhaps without clothing, or only half clad.

I would give the Commissioners more authority in county asylums, also: at present they have little, if any; their recommendations as to enlargement and alterations of buildings, and as to treatment, ought to be respected. Buildings already too large ought not to be made larger, contrary to their expressed and written opinions, as in the case of the Hanwell and Colney Hatch Asylums, which are to be augmented at a cost of 70,000*l*. They ought to have the appointment and discharge of the medical officers, or at all events such appointments and discharges ought not to be valid until confirmed by them. No poor-law medical appointments or discharges are valid without the consent of the Commissioners; why should it not be so with lunacy appointments? If the plan works well in the one case, doubtless it would in the other. The medical superintendent of a lunatic asylum ought to be in a more independent position than he is at present; it is quite impossible to please so many masters, and if his views do not coincide with all, he has enemies, and ultimately gets dismissed. In the discharge of Mr Miller, late superintendent of the Bucks County Lunatic Asylum, the Magistrates actually refused to give their reason for dismissing him. The medical superintendent ought to have the appointment of all the subordinate officers and servants.

4. With regard to the curability of insanity, there can be no doubt that if persons were sent to an asylum immediately on the disease making its appearance, that from fifty to seventy per cent. would be cured. We have ample proof of this in the returns of Bethlem and St Luke's Hospitals, into which, with few exceptions, recent cases only are received. This fact cannot be too strongly impressed upon the public, inasmuch as the retaining of such patients at home for any length of

time presents an almost insurmountable obstacle to the cure of the disease.

The following table forcibly illustrates the advantages of early treatment.

Duration of Attack on admission.	Recovered Cases.	Per centage.
Under one month - - - -	504	56.250
Between one and three months -	192	21.428
Between three and six months -	94	10.491
Between six and twelve months -	50	5.580
Between one and two years - -	36	4.018
Upwards of two years - - -	20	2.232
Totals - - -	896	100.

The above cases were under treatment in County Asylums. Taking the average per-centage of recoveries at 36, the number under treatment would be 2,500. The proportion of acute cases to chronic, is as one to three.

With females insanity is much more curable than with males, and the mortality is not near so high. The next table shows the result of treatment as extracted from the annual reports of twenty public asylums. In three the recoveries of males and females not being distinguished, the information upon this point is confined to seventeen. It would very much facilitate statistical inquiry, if the Reports of all our asylums contained annually a statement of the admissions, recoveries, and deaths, and the number resident on the first of January, distinguishing the males from the females, from their

opening. Every report should also contain a table
giving the duration of attack in each case prior to
admission.

Number of Patients under Treatment.		Per-centage of Recoveries.		Number of Patients under Treatment.		Per-centage of Deaths.*	
Males.	Females.	Males.	Females.	Males.	Females.	Males.	Females.
10,007	7,382	34.93	41.63	12,633	10,162	24.64	19.20

* The per-centage of deaths in this Table has been taken upon the
admissions, and not upon the numbers resident, or under treatment in
each year.

5. In most, if not all, of the asylums in which
non-restraint has been adopted, the proportion of
recoveries has increased, whilst at the same time
the number of deaths has also proportionably diminished. (See comparative Tables at the end of this
sketch.) In the Surrey County Asylum the recoveries
from 1850 to 1855, were, males, 37.14 per cent.,
females, 47.66 per cent.; whilst during a similar period,
viz.: from 1844 to 1849, prior to the introduction of
non-restraint, they only amounted to males, 23.51 per
cent., females, 20.84 per cent. Thus in the male department there was an increase in favour of non-
restraint of 13.63 per cent., and in the female, of 26.82
per cent.; a result highly satisfactory, and reflecting
great credit on the officers, more particularly on Dr
Diamond, the Superintendent of the female department.
The mortality at this asylum was, during the first-
named period, males, 11.48, and females, 5.37 per cent.,
and during the latter period, males, 11.42, females,

7.53. At the Hanwell Asylum, the per-centage of recoveries from 1831 to December, 1840 was, males, 24.92, females, 23.97, and since that period, to December, 1855, it has been, males, 22.81, females, 27.87, giving a slight increase in favour of non-restraint, whilst the mortality is largely in its favour. Deaths per cent. during the restraint period, males, 55.11, females, 49.90; during the non-restraint period, males, 28.31, females, 16.34. At the Norfolk Asylum, which has been notorious for the amount of restraint employed there, and for its mis-management (the Superintendent being a layman, formerly an attendant of the Hanwell Asylum), the deaths from 1814 to December 31, 1852, were, males, 43.08 per cent., females 36.38,* whilst during the year 1853, when Dr Foote acted as Physician (though not allowed to take the superintendence), and the non-restraint system was fully carried out, the result was, recoveries, males, 47.22 per cent., females, 46.80: deaths, males, 10.85, females, 8.25. The *first* report of this institution, established in 1814, was published by Dr Foote in 1854. That gentleman had brought the asylum into a creditable state; he had improved the dietary, had introduced various amusements and recreations, and effected great changes. But his improved treatment of the patients was attended with expense, and was not in accordance with the views of the visitors, and the narrow-minded policy of the super-

---

* The per-centage of deaths of the Hanwell and Norfolk Asylums, during the restraint period, has been taken upon the admissions, and not upon the numbers under treatment in each year, as in the comparative Tables. The numbers under treatment, and the recoveries at the latter asylum were not easily ascertainable.

intendent, and consequently he was dismissed. The salary of the physician at the Norfolk Asylum is 100*l.* per annum. How degrading to think, that the services of that officer should be computed at such a miserable pittance, and that he should occupy a subordinate position in the control and management of the institution! I regret to observe that in many of our lunatic asylums the remuneration of the medical officers is simply on a par with that of the Matron. No medical officer should receive less than 300*l.* per annum, and the salary should range from 300*l.* to 500*l.*, according to the size of the building. Lunatic asylums should not in any case be built to accommodate more than 500 patients. The gigantic size of some of our asylums militates strongly against their success, the mortality when such numbers of patients are congregated together being, I had almost said, necessarily large.

6. The non-restraint system has been attacked by some as substituting " concealed severity " for " mechanical restraint." I fear there was infinitely more " concealed severity " in the palmy days of the strait-waistcoat, than could possibly co-exist with the system of surveillance, and the free admission of the public to these institutions. When I delivered my Lecture in 1838, I stated that its object was " to advocate the total abolition," not only of mechanical restraint, but " of every species and degree of severity, as applied to patients in our asylums." Every deviation from this principle should be immediately checked, and the utmost care be taken that no abuse whatever shall creep in; that neither unnecessary force, nor drugs, nor the

douche, nor the bath of surprise, nor prolonged shower or other baths, be employed, as substitutes for mechanical restraint. *They form no part of the system of non-restraint*, and are essentially contrary to its first principles. Neither, on the other hand, must we be deterred by unfounded accusations from the application of proper remedies to insane, any more than to sane patients. There can be no doubt that baths, judiciously applied, are very useful, in allaying irritation, and procuring sleep; especially the warm and shower-bath together. The plan usually adopted by myself, and one which I have found most effective, is to immerse the body in warm water in one of the ordinary baths, and then, having a vessel of cold water at hand, to apply it to the head by means of the hand shower-bath. In this way you may apply any quantity of water without danger to the patient, or without occasioning pain; and you can regulate the height of the bath according to the strength of the patient. The system of prolonged shower-baths, as practised on the male side of the Surrey Asylum, and now sanctioned by the Visiting Magistrates of that institution, is most dangerous, as well as barbarous and cruel, and ought to be put a stop to. No person even in robust health could afford the loss of so much animal heat as would be the result of twenty minutes', or half an hour's exposure to the effects of a shower-bath thus prolonged. The shock is immense, the pain exquisite; and to follow up this with a dose of emetic tartar, is almost certain to bring about a fatal termination.

While upon this subject I beg leave again emphatically to deny that shower-baths are devices made use of in lunatic asylums under the present system, instead of chains, and other modes of restraint.* Shower-baths were employed long before the introduction of non-restraint, and were as much used in former days as now. No one can have a greater horror of the douche, or of prolonged shower-baths, than myself, and under no circumstances would I sanction their employment. That the patient Dolly, of the Surrey Asylum, referred to by the Recorder and Dr Christison, died from the effects of the shower-bath, and the dose of tartar emetic subsequently administered, there cannot be a doubt; and the public ought to be much indebted to the Commissioners in Lunacy for the steps taken by them in the matter. Dr Diamond, in giving his evidence, stated, " that the condition of the body very much astonished

---

* Extract from the Recorder's address to the Grand Jury at the Central Criminal Court, July 7, 1856, as reported in the ' Times,' July 8 :—" It appeared that the patient, who was an old man, sixty-five years of age, had been subjected to a shower-bath; which was one of the devices made use of under the present system in lunatic asylums, instead of chains and other modes of restraint, that were formerly employed for the purpose of lowering the patients, and which he believed had been found beneficial."

From Dr Christison's letter to Dr Bence Jones :—" I presume that, as usual in cases of this kind, there will be no want of asylum attendants of all degrees to testify that the treatment in question is good, efficacious, and safe treatment for a refractory patient of sixty-five years of age. But, for my part, I must own to having felt surprise, as Professor of Materia Medica, to find that the protracted use of the shower-bath was thought admissible as a remedy, and no less astonished to learn, as a philanthropist, that such discipline formed anywhere a part of the boasted non-restraint system in the management of the insane."

him—it was as white as marble—it was like a piece of alabaster." In truth, the continued application of cold to the surface of the body threw the blood inwards, and so distended the heart, that it became paralysed, and death was the result. The distention of the heart will account for its *apparently* diseased state, for upon more minute examination it proved to be perfectly healthy. The bath was of twenty-eight minutes' duration, and 618 gallons of water was the quantity used upon the occasion.

7. In the Lecture delivered in 1838, I had laid it down as an axiom, that "in the treatment of the insane, medicine is of little avail, except (of course) when they are suffering also from other diseases, to which lunatics, as well as sane persons, are liable." "*Moral treatment, with a view to induce habits of self-control, is all and everything.*" This principle, understood as I intended it, I believe to be, on the whole, correct : but the exception is more frequent than I then thought. The connection of insanity with an excited state of the nerves and brain, which are bodily organs, is so intimate, that if these can be soothed, the mind is also calmed. My opinion, I confess, is somewhat modified by this consideration, and by the experience since acquired. Therefore I hesitate not to avow the conviction that whilst much must ever depend on the latter, the former is a very useful adjunct, and for this reason :—that in most cases of insanity, there is more or less derangement of some bodily organ or function. I have frequently found opiates very useful, particularly henbane, com-

bined with the compound spirit of sulphuric ether;
the acetate and muriate of morphia, and the sedative
solution of opium (Battley's). In cases of maniacal
excitement, Battley's solution, with small doses of
tartar emetic, is exceedingly effective and safe. Tonics
also are very useful, and sometimes stimulants. There
are cases in which stimulants cannot be dispensed with.
The insane should live well, and be well clothed,
particularly in winter. In many chronic cases, particularly where there is a contracted state of the pupils,
the bichloride of mercury given in small doses, and
the treatment persisted in for some time, will be found
efficacious. I had lately a gentleman under my care
whose case was considered helpless;—he had been
more than twelve months insane, and had epileptic
fits, and at times was very violent and dangerous. In
this case, the 12th of a grain was given three times
a day, with ten minims of the compound spirit of
sulphuric ether, and one ounce of decoction of bark;
—a blister was applied to the back of his neck, and
kept open for several days;—a generous diet was
allowed, for his circulation was languid, and with this
treatment kept up for a few weeks he recovered, and
has remained well ever since, now nearly twelve months.
In this patient there was a great tendency to suicide,
and he required constant watching. He occasionally
refused food, and took no notice of surrounding objects.
He had not been under medical treatment many days
before a decided change for the better was observed.
He soon entered into conversation, became very com-
municative, and cards and bagatelle were favourite

amusements with him. He was sent out several times in the carriage, once to the Crystal Palace, and on another occasion to town. He was very industrious during the period of his convalescence, working for hours in the hay-field, and assisting the men in stacking.

8. The padded room is found exceedingly effective in cases where patients are bent upon injuring themselves by knocking their heads against the wall: and the poor epileptic, formerly fastened to his bedstead, is now provided with a sleeping-room, the walls of which are padded from the floor to about four feet in height. It is very seldom necessary to resort to seclusion, although in some cases, for short periods, I have seen very good effects arise from its use; and a darkened room is occasionally very beneficial, particularly in cases of acute mania.

For patients who destroy their clothes strong plaid dresses are provided, with the under-clothing made of twilled linen. The blankets at night are encased in plaid ticking, and strongly quilted. The bed and pillows are also enclosed, and the sheets are of strong twilled linen. For patients who undress themselves, screw buttons, and hooks and eyes which fasten with a key, have been provided; and these are also used for keeping on boots. List shoes are worn by patients who kick. Care should be taken to keep the finger-nails of dangerous and destructive patients closely cut, because with the nail a deal of mischief may be effected, and violent females are particularly apt to use their nails in attacking others. Never allow a patient to see that you feel afraid—once show fear, and you have no longer any control. When a patient requires food to be forcibly administered, I prefer the use of a feeder, resembling a wine-funnel with a stop-cock attached to it. The food is introduced through the nostril. There is no doubt that the forcible introduction of the stomach-pump, in the case of a patient struggling violently against it, is attended with danger; the coats of the stomach being liable to structural injury, which may, and I believe has in some instances, actually occasioned death.

9. The condition of the lunatic prior to the introduction of non-restraint may be gathered from the following extracts.

From the Report of the Lancaster Asylum for 1841 :

"From the opening of this Asylum in the year 1816, mechanical restraint appears to have been extensively employed; and at the time your officers took charge they found twenty-nine persons wearing either handcuffs, leg-locks, or strait-waistcoats— exclusive of between thirty and forty patients who were chained down during the day-time on seats so constructed as to answer all the purposes of water-closets, in rooms known by the appellation of ' the warm-rooms:' moreover, during the night-time all the epileptic and violent patients were chained or otherwise secured in bed. It was also an established custom to place every case on admission under restraint during the night-time, for a longer or a shorter period, as might appear expedient. Before proceeding any further it may be advisable, more espe-

cially as some erroneous statements have already
appeared about these 'warm-rooms,' to give a general
idea of their construction and situation. They are two
in number, one for the females and the other for the
males, situated in the centre of the building in juxta-
position, and obtain their designation from the circumstance of the floors, which are of stone, being heated by
flues. They are thirty-four feet long by eighteen broad,
and fourteen feet high; and, although they are dark and
gloomy in their appearance, they are tolerably well
ventilated. Along the inner wall of these rooms were
placed fourteen stalls or boxed seats answering the
double purpose, as stated above, of seats and water-
closets; and at the end of each room three similar seats,
not answering the purpose of water-closets, were affixed.
Idiotic and violent patients, and those of filthy habits,
were chained in these seats from early in the morning
until bed-time: the men were clothed in a short petticoat; and, owing to the floor being warmed, neither the
men nor women were usually allowed shoes or stockings.
A long leaden trough, immediately below these seats and
communicating with a common drain or sewer, was
repeatedly washed out during the day by turning on a
tap of water at the upper part."

From the Report of the Northampton Asylum
for 1839:

"The quoted statements in the following cases are
by the resident officer of the institution from which the
patients were removed:—

" 'J. S.—Subject to epileptic fits, very violent and

malicious, will fight, kick, and bite; not to be trusted with any safety to the attendants.

" ' S. L.—In every respect as bad as J. S., but *worse if possible.'*

" When these men were admitted, *their legs were confined by heavy irons, which barely allowed one foot to be shuffled a few inches before its fellow; and their wrists by figure-of-8 handcuffs.* The son of the officer refused to take these instruments away with him, upon learning that we were unprovided with substitutes; declaring that he should consider himself personally answerably for our lives, were the patients set at liberty.

" ' S. M.—Violent and dangerous to the attendants; has never yet been without personal restraint (fifty-nine weeks), destroys her clothes, and is very dirty and obscene.'

" *Her legs were confined by irons, precisely similar to those in cases J. S. and S. L.; but the hands were fastened by handcuffs, behind her back.*

" ' T. H., described as exceedingly dangerous, having so frequently made violent and wanton attacks on the keepers, that it was unsafe to leave him *one moment* unrestrained.'

" The removal of this man and his fellow-sufferers (seven in number) arose out of the representations made by the parochial officers, who visited him at his previous place of confinement. These individuals stated to the local authorities *that they found him in a state of nudity; lying on wet and dirty straw, chained by one wrist and ankle to the bedstead, and that from the appearance of* *his person, apartment, and bed, they conceived that the two former could not have been cleansed, or the latter exchanged, for some length of time : and also, that it was necessary to empty his mouth* by means of a spoon and some water, before he could reply to their questions.*

"S. T., when brought to the asylum, *was restrained by a strait-waistcoat: on examining his person, it was discovered to be literally black from bruises in every part excepting the face. His wrists and ankles were excoriated and ulcerated by the pressure of ligatures, and the backs of his hands were much contused.* He was extremely exhausted; the moment an attendant appeared, he became excited, called upon us to turn him out of the room, and lock him up; attempted to effect this object himself, and begged of us, *most piteously*, not to leave him alone with the keeper, as he was sure he should be ' *murdered.*' This conduct being always repeated under similar circumstances, a convalescent private patient volunteered to take charge of him, and he has since been much more tranquil. * * * Why was the presence of the attendant so hateful and terrible to him? Because the strait-waistcoat and the tying-down in bed, had previously afforded an ' irritable, revengeful, and selfish ' keeper the opportunity to multiply his physical sufferings by blows, *which the coward could never have dared to inflict, had his victim possessed the power to retaliate!* Those who are practically acquainted with the doings of a lunatic ward, must corroborate the assertion, *if they will but be sincere, that the fatuous, imbecile and dirty,*

---

* " Its contents can be better imagined than described."

are the usual victims of cruelty; the strong never,—
unless rendered equally helpless and unresisting by
coercion."

These patients were not subjected to any restraint
at the Northampton Asylum. J. S. became very useful
to the attendants, was allowed to have a pass-key, and
evinced great humanity towards his fellow-sufferers;
S. L. "worked at his trade as a tailor;" T. H. "very
soon became an orderly inmate;" and S. M., who had
not been without personal restraint for fifty-nine weeks,
was discharged recovered, after a sojourn of eight
months.

When Dr Conolly entered upon his duties at the
Hanwell Asylum (1839) he found about 600 instruments of restraint, half of which were leg-locks and
handcuffs. On the female side there were forty patients
who were almost always under restraint, fourteen of
them being in restraint chairs. It was usual also to
fasten the epileptics at night, exceeding one hundred in
number, by one hand to their bedsteads. At the
Surrey County Asylum, even as late as the year 1848,
no less than fifty-nine female patients out of 238
were under restraint.

In some of the licensed houses patients were habitually chained to their bedsteads, naked, with very
little covering, and some slept in hovels or outhouses,
without fire or an attendant within call. Not many
years ago I had ocular proof of this at a house near
Lichfield: the outhouses were then condemned, and the
licence, I find, has since been withdrawn. "In a house
at Fonthill, in Wiltshire, out of 14 male patients, only

one was without fetters or handcuffs."*   " In a private
asylum near London," where the " dirty patients were
chained to their cribs from Saturday night till Monday
morning, and confined without intermission 'in crowded,
ill-ventilated places,' 70 out of about 400 patients were
almost invariably in irons."   At this house the patients
slept " naked upon straw, with nothing but a blanket
to cover them, and the window was an aperture without
glass.   One towel a week was accorded for the use of
170 patients, and some were mopped with cold water,
in the severest weather "†

10. Let us see what followed the introduction of
the non-restraint system.   Instead of the monotonous
life that was customary in our asylums, we have amusements of all kinds for the patients, fêtes, and balls, and
tea-drinkings, and excursions, and even lectures and
theatrical representations.   Quiet and orderly patients
are sometimes allowed to go to the Theatres and to
Concerts; and in London and the neighbourhood, the
Crystal Palace, and British Museum, and Kew Gardens,
are favourite places of resort.   Asylums are now provided with libraries, billiard-rooms, and ball-rooms;
and the patients have the privilege of reading the daily
papers, as well as the weekly and other periodicals.
' Punch' is a great favourite with them.   We have no
longer rooms without furniture; and instead of iron
and heavy forms fastened to the ground, we have the

* ' Conolly on the Treatment of the Insane, without Mechanical
Restraints,' p. 21.
† Idem, pp. 21, 22.

ordinary house furniture, with a plentiful supply of lounging-chairs, sofas, ottomans, &c. One of the greatest improvements has been the destruction of the old iron fire-guards, which at one time were considered indispensable. These guards were heavy and cumbersome, and had to be opened whenever the fires required mending or stirring; and to carpets they were very destructive, as they moved upon casters. Like the window-guards, they were not only inconvenient, but suggestive. A patient at the Lincoln Asylum burnt himself to death, having obtained a light by introducing a piece of paper or stick between the bars, and set fire to his clothes. Subsequently the guards were lined with fine wire work. Now the fires are without guards, and yet we hear of no accidents from burning, *watchfulness being the substitute.* Indeed, when mechanical contrivances were in vogue, the patients were not always under surveillance, and this will account for broken windows, strangling in strait-waistcoats, accidents by burning, murder, &c. It is quite clear that mechanical contrivances did not prevent accidents, nor destruction to property; for with window guards, windows were broken; with fire-guards, patients were burnt to death; and with strait-waistcoats and other instruments, patients were hanged, strangled, and murdered. Of two patients, *both under restraint,* one was murdered by the other at the York Asylum. There is nothing gives to an asylum so much the appearance of home as an open fire; it is much appreciated by the patients, who sit round it, the very picture of contentment. Before the old fire-guards the patients used to crouch in abject misery. Then, again, out of doors, we have flowers, and shrubs, and ornamental walks; here may be seen a tent with coloured flags flying from each end, or from the centre;—there a statue,—in another part a fountain,—and further on a conservatory:—then there are fowls, and chickens, and pigeons, and guinea-pigs, distributed in different parts of the grounds, and games are provided, such as cricket, quoits, tennis, Jack's alive, and skittles. In fact nothing that could possibly amuse has been lost sight of. In pauper asylums rocking-chairs are provided for the amusement of the more dangerous patients. In those institutions, the female patients are very much employed in the cleaning of the establishment, in cooking, washing, and in the making up of clothes, and keeping them in repair; and the males in gardening and farm-work. Shoemaking is much followed in some institutions, but I disapprove of it, in consequence of the dangerous nature of the tools required in this sedentary, and often *solitary* occupation. At the Wakefield Asylum, under the superintendence of the late Sir William Ellis, an attendant was killed by a patient who was so employed, and who up to that period had been considered harmless. The upper classes are more devoted to recreations than to useful employment; but the ladies do a great deal of fancy and ornamental work, and are generally industrious. A piano in a lady's sitting-room is a great source of amusement. Then, again, as to meals: formerly the meat was cut up for all the patients, now the greater part are provided with knives and forks, and spoons, so that they can really enjoy their food. They have no longer the tin can, but cups and saucers, and tea-pots, and even kettles are introduced. It is now a pleasure to see them at their meals. Not many years ago they used to swallow food after the fashion of wild animals; sometimes they were very voracious, and would cram as much into their mouths as possible, and were in danger of being choked. Now they are carefully watched, and if a patient is disposed to be voracious, he is taught to be moderate. A patient thus treated soon learns to control himself.

I may here remark that it is a most gratifying sight to observe the patients attending, as they do now, in all our asylums, the celebration of divine worship on Sundays. Many of them join in the singing, and conduct themselves well throughout the service. In all well-regulated institutions there are daily morning and evening prayers. The celebration of the Holy Communion, however, seems to me a glaring impropriety. I consider that if a patient is in a suitable state of mind to receive the Sacrament, he is fit to be discharged.

The galleries of our public asylums are fitted up with aviaries—plants are distributed in the windows—the walls are covered with pictures, and works of art; statues and statuettes are to be seen in almost all parts of the building. This is the case at Bethlem, and the change has been effected there by the exertions of the able and talented Physician and Superintendent, Dr Hood. I recollect Bethlem as a mere pest-house, when a sight of the patients struck one with terror. The court-yards, now laid out as pleasure-grounds, used to be covered with gravel, and here and there was a strong seat fastened to the ground, with a patient chained to it by the leg. The only drawback to Bethlem is the male criminal wing, which is indeed a remnant of bygone ages. Balls are held once a week, and the billiard-room is open until a certain hour in the evening, when the gas is put out, and the patients retire for the night.

I have had frequent opportunities of seeing the interior of the Surrey County Asylum (Female department), under the Superintendence of Dr Diamond, whose exertions in behalf of the insane have been most praiseworthy. Great changes have been effected there by him. Although a pauper establishment, the patients have every comfort; and pictures, and plants, and books abound for their amusement. The doctor's approach is evidently hailed with delight. I was present at one of their out-door fêtes about two or three years ago; and a most animated scene it was. I cannot say whether the music, or the dancing, or the strawberries and cream, were enjoyed most; but certain it is that a very agreeable afternoon was spent, not only by the patients, but by the visitors. Dr Diamond has for some time been engaged in taking a series of photographic portraits, illustrating the effects of insanity upon the expression and countenance. He has divided these into three distinct periods, as regards each individual, viz.: the period of the paroxysms, or the date of the most aggravated symptoms: the period of partial recovery, and that of complete restoration. It is evident that such illustrations form a very valuable adjunct to the study of insanity; and it is only under the system of non-restraint that they can be depended upon; inasmuch as formerly these portraits could only delineate the effects of insanity, aggravated by the various modes of restraint, terror, and ill-usage of the patient then resorted to, and the consequent permanent feelings of hatred and revenge thence arising: in a word, they served to illustrate the effects of the treatment, rather than the malady itself, as is sufficiently apparent in the work of Sir Alexander Morison, although entitled ' The Physiognomy of Mental Diseases." Dr Diamond's labours therefore are exceedingly valuable, and will be appreciated in proportion as they are known.

I had lately an opportunity of visiting St Luke's Hospital, accompanied by the Medical officer, Mr Stevens. The improvements in the building itself had not kept pace with the improved system of treatment. The wards had been divided, the centre of the building had been modernised, but the other parts remained unaltered, and were greatly deficient in comfort and cleanliness, having all the appearance of an old-fashioned prison. The walls had not been coloured for some time, and the wash, perhaps for want of glue, came off upon the patients' clothes, and gave them a very unsightly and slovenly appearance. The attendants had a singular aspect, the men wearing white aprons, and both men and women having long chains with the keys suspended from them. Even in the modernised part of the building the fire-places were guarded. The airing courts are dismal and cramped; in fact, the site is not at all suited for such an institution, as it scarcely admits of improvements. The old plunge-bath was still in use.

11. In France the old system is still adhered to. At this time French "Aliénistes" cry down non-restraint, as the English physicians used to do in the earlier years of its existence. It would appear from a statement made by Dr H. Van Leeuwen, of Jersey, that they condemn the system without knowing anything about it, and make charges against it without even troubling themselves to ascertain whether there be any foundation for such charges; for instance, they assert we have always our patients in seclusion. Now it is well known that seclusion is so seldom resorted to, that twelve months will pass by, even in our largest asylums, without any instance of its employment: that when used it is merely remedial, and for short periods only. In the Lincoln Asylum it has for some years been dispensed with altogether. In the days of restraint it was largely employed in conjunction with chains; but it was necessary then, and not a word was heard of its impropriety. I am glad to observe, that in the Annual Reports of the Colney Hatch and Surrey County Asylums, tables are given containing the several instances of seclusion employed throughout the year. This example might be followed with advantage by other asylums.

Monsieur Moreau de Tours asserts, that non-restraint is " an idea entirely Britannic, an impossibility in most cases, an illusion always, the expression itself a lie."

During the summer of 1855, I had an opportunity of inspecting the two large asylums at Paris, the Bicêtre, and Saltpêtrière, the former for male, and the latter for female lunatics. I was accompanied by a friend. The Bicêtre contained (July 4, 1855), 850 patients, the Saltpêtrière 1,300. The patients are divided into sections; the Bicêtre had three, and the Saltpêtrière five. We were only permitted to see one section in each asylum. The sections were subdivided into three classes. The camisole (strait-waistcoat) was in general use, as well as the old restraint-chairs; in many cases both being employed at the same time. The stench from the patients using the chairs was intolerable. Many of the patients were only half clad, and very dirty, whilst some of the men wore petticoats, and one I observed in a state of nudity, his skin scorched by the burning sun. The attendant who accompanied us through the wards stated that the camisole was employed to prevent patients from tearing their clothes, and from scratching themselves, and it was worn at night by the violent and mischievous patients. The violent patients at the Saltpêtrière slept in detached buildings, fourteen of which I observed in one court-yard. These buildings consisted of a single room with a heavy sliding door, and the window had heavy iron stanchions with shutters, but were not glazed. There were no means of heating these buildings. At the Bicêtre the rooms for such patients were similar in appearance, but not detached; the windows were also unglazed. Here they had a warming apparatus. I was told at the Saltpêtrière, that the *douche* was used as a punishment, whilst at the Bicêtre the attendant, upon being asked the question, answered in the negative. In the latter institution the *douche* was placed above the ordinary bath, and one of the patients

was ready to show us its use. I saw three patients in
the bath; they remain in for very long periods. The
patient whilst using the bath is locked in it, the head
being fixed in a sheet of iron which covers the upper
third of the bath, and through the centre of which
there is a hole. It was a most disgusting sight: the
poor fellows jabbered, and distorted their faces, and
made many attempts to extricate themselves. They
looked exactly as though they had been decapitated.
If very troublesome, no doubt the *douche* above is
brought into requisition. The rotatory chair is not
used. The homicidal patients are in a separate building, circular in form, surrounded by a very high and
strong iron fence, connected with the building at the
top, so that escape is impossible. We were not allowed
to see these patients; we merely saw the building from
a distant court. The employments for the men were
said to be agricultural, 300 acres being cultivated by
150 patients. The windows were all guarded, even in
the salle-à-manger [dining hall], which contained a few
pictures and busts. The courts are planted with trees,
and some with flowers and shrubs; about 600 of the
females were said to be employed. A school has been
established more for amusement than instruction: about
a dozen male patients generally attend; a gymnasium
has been provided for the boys and idiotic patients.
Black eyes and bruised faces were rather numerous, and
strait-waistcoats were in use even amongst the ordinary
patients.

At Rouen I visited the Quartemares and St Yon
Asylums. I was accompanied over the latter institu-

tion by Drs Bouteville* and Marielle, from whom I received very kind attention. Quartemares had recently been rebuilt; some parts of it were not then finished. Both asylums had patients of the upper, as well as of the lower classes. Some of the apartments were very beautifully furnished, and the decorations had been chosen without regard to cost. There was a plentiful supply of pictures, ornamental clocks, vases, plants, flowers, &c. &c. The beds for the upper classes were elegant and light, the curtains being of embroidered muslin, suspended from a brass ring, loosely fixed to the ceiling. I was much pleased with the taste which had been displayed in the furnishing of these apartments; no comfort had been lost sight of. The airing grounds were nicely laid out, and cheerful; as usual in hot countries the trees were planted in rows, so that the patients had an opportunity of getting into the shade, a very great luxury during the summer months. Quartemares contained 386 male patients. I did not see any one under restraint in that asylum, but I was afterwards told by Dr Bouteville, the Physician to that establishment, that five patients were wearing the camisole. It was clear, therefore, that the whole of the patients had not come under my view. I counted ten patients with the strait-waistcoat on at St Yon: that asylum contained 668 females. About 250 male patients were employed at Quartemares, some on the farm,

---

* Dr Bouteville wore the Cross of the Legion of Honour. The French understand infinitely better than we do the value of such stimulants to laudable exertion. How long would Dr B. have waited in England for any such national tribute to his merits!

others in the garden, &c.; 350 females were employed at St Yon; 30 males were insensible to natural calls, and 80 females. The *douche* was employed at both asylums.

12. Although a favourable impulse has been given generally to the improved treatment of the insane, even in asylums which have not adopted the non-restraint system in its full extent, yet it is evident that the state and condition of those asylums will not bear comparison, either abroad or in this country, with that of the institutions where non-restraint is the law. The testimonies hereto annexed, as well as that of Dr Conolly before given, amply justify this assertion. And the formation of such a society as that of the Association of Medical Officers of Asylums for the Insane, cannot but contribute to the still further development of every plan essential to good management. The able and enlightened journal of that Society, edited by Dr Bucknill, is one which has done good service, both at home and abroad, and at every meeting of the Society opinions are discussed and suggestions made, all tending to one great and humane object, viz., the restoration, to their friends and to society, of thousands of our afflicted fellow-creatures, and, where this cannot be accomplished, the amelioration of their condition, the increase of their comforts, their rescue, at all events, from their state of abject misery, which was formerly their inevitable doom. Such a design is worthy of the employment of our highest faculties—of our highest zeal; and every step we take in this direction

is fraught with satisfaction to ourselves and benefit to others. This consideration alone is sufficient to stimulate and encourage our best efforts: and that such results have followed the introduction of non-restraint, there is no lack of proof. With some striking evidence on this point, I now conclude these observations.

The late T. O. Pritchard, Esq., M.D.—"I cannot quit this subject, without referring to the results of the modern system, as it relates to the patients: the directors of the Lincoln Asylum record, that 'the increased proportion of recoveries, under the full deve-lopment of the system of non-restraint, non-seclusion, and exhilarating engagement, in this house, affords gratifying assurance of the soundness of the practice; and the reduced duration, and consequently reduced cost, of the period of treatment, are conclusive as to its economy.' Dr Conolly also reports, that 'Insanity, thus treated, undergoes great if not unexpected modifications; and the wards of Lunatic Asylums no longer illustrate the harrowing description of their former state. Mania, not exasperated by severity, and melancholy, not deepened by the want of ordinary consolations, lose the exaggerated character in which they were formerly beheld. Hope takes the place of fear; serenity is substituted for discontent; and the mind is left in a condition favourable to every impression likely to call forth salutary efforts. A chance is thus afforded, to every impaired mind, of recovery to an extent only limited by causes which no human art can remove.'

" I entirely coincide with the foregoing observations. Unfortunately, however, *the majority of cases in which the beneficial effects of humane treatment are the most conspicuous, occur in the incurable clases.* Their state on admission is rarely witnessed by any others than those resident in the Asylum; their histories, and the details of their former sufferings, are therefore known but to a few. It is, however, no uncommon circumstance to hear an idiotic female express her dread, lest the ' *head keeper* ' should come and ' *beat her,*' or to witness her delight at learning that she should sleep in a bed. She may tell you how herself, and three or four others, have long slept on a little straw, scattered over the floor of a small room, and that *every night for four years her hands had been strapped behind her, before retiring* TO REST. Several may have been brought in with contracted joints, from continued confinement in strait-waistcoats, or from being fastened to their cribs. And another may be reported to have been ' *bricked up in a recess ;*' she may not be able to bear the irritation produced by her clothing, and have no power to signify her wants, than by the utterance of a few unintelligible sounds. *Yet many thus admitted, are now the most quiet, industrious, and useful of our inmates.* Scars may, nevertheless, be still discovered on their ankles and wrists, and a slight halt may be detected in their gait, when the attention of the visitor is excited; but they do not add to the per-centage of our recoveries, though *the degree of improvement that has been effected, is comparatively greater than ever takes place in the convalescence of a recent case.* The benevolent intentions of the founders of this institution have not however been less completely, though less palpably, carried into effect."—Fourth Annual Report, Northampton Asylum, 1841-2, pp. 67, 68.

Patrick Nimmo, Esq., M.D., and T. T. Wingett, Esq., M.D.—" The number discharged recovered has been 60 per cent. of the cases admitted.

" The number of deaths has been 4·85 per cent. of the daily averaged number of patients resident. No serious accident has occurred.

" *These figures amply testify that the system of treatment pursued has been blessed with good results;* and encourage perseverance in the course hitherto pursued.

" The moral or administrative aspect of an Asylum is that feature in its character which chiefly determines its reputation. If carefully cultivated and watched, an Asylum assumes one of the most interesting objects for our regard ; while, on the other hand, the want of a just appreciation of its power and influence, either for good or ill, induces inevitable deformity and disappointment. Herein consists the main difference between the past and mistaken, and the present and enlightened methods, which has converted an Asylum from a scene in which a cursory visit revealed nothing save what was extreme and extraordinary in calamity, to a scene in which nothing extraordinary is visible; and which has accordingly made a well-regulated Asylum cease to be an object of

interest for idle curiosity. Upon passing through the
wards of the most excitable patients, the disappearance
of all means of mechanical restraint suggests to the
inexperienced the question—' Are these really the most
dangerous class of lunatics?' Happily, in proportion
as external and avoidable irritations have ceased to be
added to those existing within the patient, the humili-
ating aspects of the disease have diminished; comfort
and composure have been augmented; and, as an obvious consequence, the malady rendered more amenable
to medical treatment."—Thirty-second Annual Report
of the Dundee Royal Asylum for Lunatics, 1853,
pp. 17, 18.

" The main principles of the regime of this Institution have been established for many years; and the
efforts of every succeeding year have been directed
to their more complete and extended application.
Since 1842 there has been an entire disuse of all
articles for mechanically restraining the limbs of
patients ; and every available and justifiable method
has been adopted for making the contrast between the
customs and amenities of ordinary society, and the
discipline established, as narrow and as little irksome
as possible. This regime has been examined by the
present illustrious Chairman of the Lunacy Commission
of England, the Earl of Shaftesbury, who expressed
his approbation of what he characterized as the
' humane system' pursued.

" This regime recognizes the fact that, when an
individual crosses the threshold of an Asylum, he does
not necessarily surrender all his freedom of action,

nor is he expected to renounce all the tastes and habits which have ministered to his happiness in other days. His freedom and his pleasure are curtailed only in that precise measure which are imperatively demanded as essential to safety or cure. The inmate of an Asylum has his recognised and legitimate rights, and his curator has corresponding duties, and if these rights are unrecognised and these duties neglected the patient is persecuted or tyrannized over. If a wish be expressed or a demand made, either the point at issue must be conceded, or the refusal must be based upon reasonable and conscientious considerations. Arbitrary authority must be scrupulously prevented from assuming the position of necessary and judicious treatment and discipline. It is the minority only of the inmates of an Asylum in whom the mind is totally wrecked or obscured. The majority can think, and feel, and act, within a limited sphere, precisely as they were accustomed to do before infirmity assailed them. The extraordinary and multifarious statements which are heard in an Asylum, during a casual visit, are apt to be considered as the common and only characteristic of the minds of the inhabitants. If such were really the case the labours of those upon whom devolves the management would be immensely simplified, and they would be delivered from many embarrassing and painful positions. There are, however, tongues which the casual visitor never hears; individuals whose sensitive feelings induce them to shrink away from the observation of the stranger and the inquisitive, whose perception of rectitude and honour is unimpaired, who require our attention, and whose treatment must receive the greatest delicacy, tact, and judgment, at our hands. To distinguish between the real and the simulated improvement; to detect the cunning and dexterous manœuvre under the guise of the honourable and sincere pledge; to define the limits of safety, in order to the prevention of unnecessary irritation, discomfort, and severity of discipline, are constant problems for our solution. As in society at large, so also in an insane community, duplicity in some, and truth and elevated sentiment in others are to be found, and it is one of the charms of the modern ameliorations in the management of the insane that this fact has been recognized. Routine, cold, and unsympathizing methods of management are condemned as intolerable, and the benevolent rule has been established that the insane must be treated, as nearly as is possible, like rational and responsible beings. That occasionally events will occur to disappoint and discourage is to be expected, but it is consolatory and cheering to be assured that *the abolition of the late prison-like and unconciliating discipline, which was prompted by a mistaken idea of danger, has not the effect of multiplying these.* They rarely follow the scrupulous observance of the instructions and rules prescribed.

" The number discharged recovered during the year has been 53·4 per cent. of the cases admitted. The mortality during the year has been 4·3 per cent. of the daily average number of patients resident."—Thirty-third Annual Report of the Dundee Royal Asylum, 1854, pp. 20, 21, 22.

W. Denne, Esq., Surgeon.—"The disuse of mechanical restraint has been mentioned with expressions of gratitude, by several of the poor afflicted inmates; and since I have had the charge, there has not been one case in which its use would have been justifiable. *One prominent fact connected with this subject is, that the amount of clothing destroyed has been immeasurably less than under the former system,* and at present there is not one patient in a ticking or other strong dress."—Report of Bedford County Asylum, 1854.

T. N. Brushfield, Esq., Surgeon.—"All forms of restraint have been entirely abolished; nor has there been the slightest reason to regret such a step having been taken; *it is certain that its disuse has had a beneficial effect on the minds of those patients who, at any time, had been the subjects of it.*"—Chester County Asylum, Report for 1854.

"*The treatment of the patients on the non-restraint system has been persevered in with the best possible effects.*"—Report for 1855.

R. Lloyd Williams, Esq., M.D., and G. T. Jones, Esq., Surgeon.—"Ever since the opening of the asylum in 1848, we have never had cause to deviate from the uniform and consistent practice of avoiding the slightest mechanical restraint in the treatment of the insane.

"We have sedulously endeavoured to impress upon our attendants that they are never to exhibit the slightest exhibition of temper, or resentment, for conduct however violent or provoking, and that they are to practise ' the law of kindness,' as the code by which the confidence of their patients is to be gained, and their violence subdued. The insane, on their part, with the instinctive perception so remarkable in most of them, very soon discover from the demeanour of their attendants that nothing but kind and gentle treatment only is to be used towards them; *we find that the most violent on admission very speedily become trustful; resistance ceases, and tranquillity follows, as a matter of course."*— Eighth Report of Commissioners in Lunacy, Appendix (G.), p. 124.

" *We find exercise in the open air the best sedative, in promoting sleep and tranquillity—even during the most violent maniacal paroxysms.*"—Denbigh County Lunatic Asylum, Report for 1854.

J. Hitchman, Esq. M.D.—" Since the year 1843, I have not sanctioned the use of any kind of mechanical appliance to control the limbs of any refractory or suicidal patients, and I have not met with any case in which, with good attendants, and a well-arranged building, restraint appeared necessary; on the contrary, *patients have been brought to the various institutions which have been under my care, who had been rendered more violent, and more suicidal by the means taken to control them prior to admission.*"—Eighth Report of Commissioners, Appendix (G), p. 125.

J. C. Bucknill, Esq., M.D.—" The abolition of restraint was an indispensable starting-point for efficient reform, since its employment was combined with a multitude of evils, which its removal rendered intolerable. Under restraint, the management of the insane could be conducted by a small number of attendants, without calling upon them to exercise either self-control, intelligence, or humanity; there was little need of medical skill, or employment, or recreation; it was found that the easiest plan of controlling the lunatic was by appeals to his lowest motives, especially to the most debasing of all motives, to fear.

" Without restraint, these conditions were reversed, and, above all, it became necessary to influence and control the insane by higher and better motives. In my opinion, the essential point of difference between the old and the new systems consists in this, that under the old system the insane were controlled by appeals to the lowest and basest of the motives of human action, and under the new system they are controlled by the highest motive which in each individual case it is possible to evoke.

" The lunatic is unable, without assistance, to control his actions, so that they may tend to his own well-being, and to that of society. He is therefore placed under care and treatment, that he may be restored to the power of self-control; under care, that while this power remains impaired, he may be assisted in its exercise. This assistance may come in the shape of a strait-waistcoat, or in the fear of one; or it may come in the sense of duty imposed in the operation of a gentle but effective discipline, of honest pride, desire of approbation, or personal regard, or the still nobler sentiments of religion. The first motive, that of fear, belongs to man and the animals, and its exercise is degrading and brutalising; the latter motives are human, and humanising in their influence, and their development is the true touchstone of progress in the moral treatment of mental disease. It was the brutalising influence of fear, and the degrading sense of shame, which constituted the true *virus* of mechanical restraints."—Eighth Report of Commissioners, Appendix (G), p. 126.

J. G. Symes, Esq., Surgeon.—"None (restraint) has been used here during the past year, and I believe for many previous years. That restraint is not so obsolete out of asylums is evident from the fact that no less than three cases—two of them females—were brought here in strait-waistcoats; and one of the females had her legs so tightly bound, that the skin in several places was broken, and she was otherwise much bruised; yet she was guarded in a close fly by two stout women, and the relieving officer. *The moment she was released from these bonds, she walked into the asylum without the least attempt to injure any one.* It was many weeks before she recovered her harsh treatment. She is now progressing satisfactorily."—Dorset County Asylum, Report for 1855.

Donald Campbell, M.D.—"In the treatment of the patients in this asylum no mechanical restraint is adopted; all harsh measures of every description are not only found to be unnecessary; but are strictly prohibited among the attendants, and made the occasion of dismissal if discovered; and I feel justified in stating it as my opinion, that personal restraint is in no case necessary for the treatment of insanity in a properly-constructed asylum, and that *in all cases it is prejudicial.*

" 1st. In cases of insanity the feelings of the patient frequently become very sensitive, and the imposition

of restraint tends to injure the feelings and wound the
sense of self-respect, and when employed in the most
violent cases it is calculated to increase the excitement
and keep up the violence.

" 2nd. Next to removing any bodily disorder, and
bringing the health of the patient into the best possible
state, constant occupation and amusement afford the
most powerful means of curing and alleviating the
disease, which the use of mechanical restraints effectually excludes, as part of the treatment.

" 3rd. The result of mechanical restraint is frequently the formation of filthy habits, which form no
small aggravation of the wretched condition of the
patients.

" 4th. The system of restraint tends to render the
attendants less watchful; and, where the system exists,
not only is the attendant apt to be much more careless
about gaining the confidence of the patient, but the
latter is also much less disposed to yield his good-will to
one who day by day adjusts his straps or strait-waistcoat."— Eighth Report of Commissioners, Appendix
(G.), p. 129.

" The degree of personal liberty which the patients
have been permitted to enjoy has been highly conducive
to their cure.

" In no case during the year has mechanical
restraint been adopted, nor has it ever been found
necessary.

" The time is happily gone by when it was thought
enough to prevent the patient from doing violence to
himself, or those around him, by placing him in
restraint.

" No longer condemned to drag out a miserable existence in solitude and wretchedness, and frequently in chains, the spirit of the times now respects the feelings of the unhappy sufferer, fans the latent spark of reason in his mind, soothes him under the strongest excitements, and by means gentle and humane, either *restores him to himself and his home, or renders him as comfortable as possible in his unhappy state.*"—Essex County Lunatic Asylum, Report for 1855.

Edward D. De Vitre, Esq., M.D., and J. Broadhurst, Esq., Surgeon.—" It will be within the recollection of many of the visitors, that previous to the year 1840 mechanical restraint formed the rule of practice rather than the exception; all cases were on admission at night placed under restraint, and were only released when, from familiarity with their symptoms, it was thought they could be trusted without; two large compartments in the Asylum were fitted up with a variety of mechanical contrivances for the constant restraint of refractory patients. These compartments contained a row of stalled seats, surrounding nearly two-thirds of the wall in each room, and served the double purpose of a water-closet and ordinary seat; the flagged floors were heated by hot air; and the patients were secured by hand-locks to each side of the upper portion of the stalls, and by leg-locks to the lower portion, the heated floor superseding the necessity of stockings and shoes; all the bedsteads, and many of the fixed seats, were so constructed as readily to admit of the free use of mechanical means to restrain their occupants. Early in the spring of 1840 an attempt was made to mitigate the horrors of such a mode of treatment; and with the

cordial sanction and approbation of the visiting magistrates, these compartments were speedily abolished,
along with all other forms of mechanical restraint then
in common use in all parts of the establishment. Since
the above period upwards of 3,000 patients have been
under treatment, and only in one instance has it been
deemed necessary to have recourse to mechanical restraint; this occurred in 1844, in the case of a violent
epileptic patient, who was placed under restraint for a
period of six hours, the particulars of which were fully
set forth in the Report of that year; and it is gratifying to add that in no one case subsequently has it
been considered necessary or justifiable to adopt any
kind of mechanical restraint as a remedial agent. . . . *An
appeal can now be made to the statistics of the Asylum,
in proof of the unspeakable advantages of moral over
mechanical means of treatment, as observable in the
general quietness and decorum of the establishment, in the
cheerful aspect of the patients, in the comparative freedom from acts of destructive violence,. and in the large
proportion of inmates who are constantly engaged in some
useful occupation; to which might be added, a decreased
mortality, and an increased per-centage of cures.*"—Lancaster County Lunatic Asylum, Report for 1855.

Edward Palmer, Esq., M.D.—" So far as the experience of ·the superintendent of this Asylum goes,
he is convinced that *no more pernicious agents were ever
introduced into institutions for the insane than mechanical
contrivances to check the disorderly outbursts of maniacal
excitement, or to antagonise the suicidal impulses of
melancholy.* Whatever the effects of such rude means

may be on some rare and exceptional cases, whether productive of injury or otherwise, he has no doubt that their effects on the patients generally are to excite perversity and resistance to moral control, and on the attendants to inculcate a reliance on coercive measures rather than on those of a guiding and directing character. None of the presumed exceptional cases have as yet appeared in this Asylum, nor has any instrument of restraint ever been within its walls, save to call for the pleasing duty of immediately removing it from the person of some newly-arrived patient, and sending it away."—Lincolnshire County Lunatic Asylum, Report for 1855.

J. S. Allen, Esq., M.D., Monmouth Asylum.— " Mechanical restraint or coercion has not been used in any case, and the want of it has not been felt. *The general effects of non-restraint on the patients, themselves, as well as on the attendants, have been salutary.*

"Punishment of any description has been discontinued as a means of treatment, owing to its inefficiency. The plan now adopted with a violent patient is to send him or her into the garden in charge of one, or sometimes two, attendants, with directions to walk them briskly through the grounds for an hour or two, or until they complain of being tired, or show an inclination to rest. Brisk exercise in the open air has been found a valuable means of subduing excitement, as well as of procuring sleep, even after sedatives and narcotics have failed."—Eighth Report of Commissioners, Appendix (G), p. 134.

R. Foote, Esq., M.D., Norfolk County Asylum.—

"I have never seen mechanical restraint produce any beneficial effect in the treatment of mental diseases, but have seen many cases greatly relieved by the removal of restraint."—Eighth Report of Commissioners, Appendix (G), p. 134.

M. N., Bower, Esq., M.D.—" The total absence of all coercion, and the undeviating system of kindness and conciliation pursued for some years in this Asylum, and indeed in most others of recent date, *have fully justified the benevolent efforts of those philanthropists who introduced these important considerations into the treatment of the insane;* at times temporary seclusion from other patients during paroxysms of excitement may be not only necessary but even highly beneficial. Still *great would be the responsibility and severe the blame due to any one, who having witnessed the effects of the present humane system, should resort, even in one single case, to the former debasing and unnecessary use of cruelty and restraint* "—Staffordshire County Asylum,Report for 1855.

James Wilkes, Esq., Commissioner in Lunacy, late Medical Superintendent of the Staffordshire County Asylum.—" Previous to the year 1841, when I was appointed to the office I now hold in this institution, mechanical restraint was part of the system of treatment habitually employed, and its disuse was looked upon as absurd and chimerical. *Although the registers certainly show a gradual diminution of restraint for some previous years, its amount at the time referred to was considerable, and probably more than was recorded.*

" The means of restraint employed were the leather muff and wrist-straps, iron handcuffs, long leather

H

sleeves, hobbles for the legs, the restraint-chair, and various devices, specially adapted to the peculiar propensities and habits of the patients. Many of these were employed both by day and night, and, in addition, many of the patients were confined to the bedsteads by means of straps passing through iron loops.

" The evil of this system was not simply confined to the coercion of the patients, but the same principle pervaded the whole establishment, and the high windows partly or wholly protected by iron guards and wirework, the numerous staples in the walls of the galleries and rooms for confining patients to their seats, and the strongly-guarded fireplaces, gave a gloomy prison-like aspect to the interior of the building, which was still perpetuated ·externally by the cheerless, high-walled airing courts, mostly destitute of either trees or flowers. Above all, it was evident that the system adopted had a natural and inevitable tendency to demoralise, if not to brutalise, the attendants, and, perhaps, one of the not least important results of the disuse of restraint is, the marked effect it has had upon the feelings and conduct of the attendants themselves.

" In an old asylum, and with deep-rooted prejudices to contend against, many difficulties and much anxiety necessarily accompanies the first efforts to abolish restraint. Many patients, who had been habitually in restraint for years, were at once set at liberty; in others the process was gradual; but ultimately all instruments of restraint were collected together out of the different galleries; restraint-chairs were broken up, and at the same time windows were unblocked, guards removed, airing courts planted and improved; and in a variety of ways more humanising influences were brought into operation.

" The effect of this upon the old inmates of the Asylum was decidedly beneficial. One patient especially, who had been for some time wearing the muff and hobbles, and appeared to be falling into a state of fatuity, *rapidly improved upon being set at liberty, and ultimately recovered.* The excitement of the patients generally was decidedly diminished; they were less noisy at night, and, though many had become inveterately dirty in their habits, *a gradual improvement took place also in this respect.* With greater opportunities of doing mischief, less absolutely occurred; and now, without a window in the Asylum in any way protected, there is probably less breakage of glass than there formerly was. The experience of more than 12 years, during which upwards of 1,300 cases have been admitted, only tends to strengthen and confirm the opinion that, as a general rule, restraint is unnecessary and injurious in the treatment of the insane."—Eighth Report of Commissioners, Appendix (G), p. 137.

H. W. Diamond, Esq., M.D., Surrey County Asylum, Female Department. — " I fully agree in the opinion of Mr R. Gardiner Hill,* that in a properly-constructed building, with a sufficient number of suitable attendants, restraint is never necessary, never justifiable, and always injurious, in all cases of lunacy

---

* A Lecture on the Management of Lunatic Asylums and the Treatment of the Insane, &c. &c., 8vo, vol., 1839, page 21.

whatever; and this is quite the reverse of my former ideas, when my knowledge of the treatment of insanity was much more limited than at the present time. I believe that any person who would now use personal restraint or coercion is unfit to have the superintendence of an Asylum.

"I have at the present time upwards of 520 female patients under my immediate charge; and during the past five years, have admitted more than 800 cases.

"In not a single instance has any restraint been used."—Eighth Report of Commissioners, Appendix (G), p. 140.

J. Thurnam, Esq., M.D., Wilts County Asylum.— "In the Wilts County Asylum, personal restraint is never resorted to, and there is literally no instrument of coercion in the institution.

"In dealing with one very painful class of cases, the suicidal, there is no doubt that *the propensity is generally aggravated by the adoption of personal restraint;* and many instances in the experience of Asylums might be quoted where suicide has been committed under the use of such means, and *even by the aid of the instruments of coercion themselves.* Incessant watchfulness during the existence of this propensity, is the only course to be adopted; and as regards the night, nothing is better than to place the patient in an associated dormitory, surrounded by those capable of exerting some control over his actions."—Eighth Report of Commissioners, Appendix (G), p. 143.

J. S. Alderson, Esq., Surgeon. — "I have much pleasure in informing you, that during the past year, I have not used personal restraint, except in one instance, and that only for eight hours, and in this case *no advantage whatever occurred from its application.*

" I beg leave most unhesitatingly to avow that I disapprove of its use; that I believe in a well-arranged Asylum it is very seldom necessary to resort to it; although from my experience in two other similar institutions, *I do not doubt its disuse to be the more humane mode of treatment.*"—West Riding of York County Lunatic Asylum, Report for 1854.

Dr Formby, Royal Lunatic Asylum, Liverpool.— " Owing to the proximity of the institution to a dense population, we are liable to the admission of many who would be detained at home were the institution more remote. Patients are frequently received labouring under acute mania, who could not well be removed to a distance; *constant watching by night and day, and mild moral treatment, have been found all that the most trying case required.* The number of attendants has been increased, night attendants employed, padded rooms and other appliances adopted, means of recreation extended, and employment, as far as practicable, provided.

" During the last few years many improvements have taken place in the furniture, &c., and the patients, however violent, have usually respected the property of the institution; and, *although the amount of glass has been nearly doubled by the extension of the windows, it is pleasing to observe that the breakage is materially less than formerly.*

" It is sometimes urged that mechanical restraint is needed where a strong propensity to suicide exists.

The restraint, to be successful, must be unremitting ; and the experience of this institution is, that *the absence of all gloomy associations is beneficial in all such cases, and that without restraint no suicide has occurred.* It is found that everything which can remove the feeling of degradation, and encourage self-respect, is calculated to further the comfort and promote the recovery of the insane."—Report of Commissioners, Appendix (G), p. 147.

H. Stevens, Esq., Surgeon, St Luke's Hospital.—" I think it right to add, that I believe the entire abolition of every kind of mechanical restraint to be the most humane, the most efficacious, and, speaking generally, the safest plan of treatment; on the whole, less liable to objection than any other, and perfectly practicable in a well-regulated and properly-conducted institution."— Eighth Report of Commissioners, Appendix (G), p. 150.

James Stocker, Esq., Surgeon, Guy's Hospital.— " All restraint has been removed (except restriction to the room of the patient on the occurrence of violent paroxysms of mania); and *this liberty has been followed by most marked improvement in the general condition and conduct of the patients,* many of whom, having previously conducted themselves with great violence, and contracted very offensive habits, have, since the adoption of the non-restraint system, been much more quiet, cleanly, and orderly."—Eighth Report of Commissioners, Appendix (G), p. 151.

W. C. Hood, Esq., M.D., Bethlem Hospital.—" No form of mechanical restraint whatever is resorted to in this hospital. The 'Non-restraint system,' as it is called, is adhered to, *because it is found to be attended with the best and happiest results;* whereas the confinement by straps, belts, or gloves rather increases the excitement, irritates the patient, reduces the necessity of vigilant personal attendance, *and not unfrequently induces chronic or permanent mania."*—Eighth Report of Commissioners, Appendix (G), p. 152.

John Kitching, Esq., The Retreat, York.—" The total or almost complete disuse of mechanical restraint and of seclusion is another important feature, as well as the greatest single improvement of the present time in the practice of Asylums. Whatever be the station assigned to it in the order of modern improvements, *no single change has brought in its train so many advantages to the insane as this.*

" If the patient be confined to the bed or chair by straps or waistcoat, it is impossible for him to attend duly to the calls of nature, and thus a familiarity with uncleanliness is established, and the sense of self-respect injured; but if the patients are afforded every opportunity of observing cleanliness and decency, and encouraged to appreciate them, a departure from them is comparatively rare."—Ibid., p. 153.

Alonzo H. Stoeker, Esq., Grove Hall Asylum, Bow. —" Since the discontinuance of restraint, the character of the Asylum has been greatly changed; acts of violence towards the attendants and other patients have been much less frequent; attempts at suicide have been of very rare occurrence, and in no instance has it been effectually carried out; there has been a less amount of destruction of property of any kind, whilst *the patients themselves have been more orderly, cheerful, and contented.*"—Ibid., p. 158.

W. F. H. Ramsey, Esq., M.D.—" From having been engaged for upwards of twelve years in the treatment of the insane, and in the management of lunatic Asylums, and from having visited and minutely examined the best Asylums in this country, as well as those on the continent, my experience and observation enable me to state, that *non-restraint, where directed under compassionate and intelligent officers, is invariably successful.* I have never myself used or advised mechanical bodily restraint, and I am convinced, that *where it is employed all moral treatment is neutralised,* and that it militates against the acquisition of the patient's confidence, which last ought to be the first endeavour of the physician who undertakes the treatment of the insane. Efficient superintendence, by means of a proper number of attendants of intelligence and respectabilty, *has always secured the comfort and cleanliness of the patients in a more satisfactory manner than under the imposition of mechanical bodily restraint;* accidents and assaults being less frequent, and the general tranquillity and order of the Asylum increased."—Ibid., p. 159.

A. J. Sutherland, Esq., M.D.—" When I was appointed to the office of Physician to St Luke's Hospital, I had all the mechanical means of restraint removed (with the exception of the restraint-chairs, which were not broken up till Dr Arlidge became Resident Superintendent, and under whose management restraint was at length entirely abandoned). I may mention that there was a poor woman, at the time I refer to, who was kept constantly under restraint, because she threatened to burn herself, and I was told that if she were released, she would attempt to sit upon the fire, and most certainly destroy herself. *I had her released from restraint, but no accident happened.* There was also a habit of entrusting the attendants with the means of restraint for the patients at night, in consequence of an accident which had occurred some years before to one of the patients; but this was dispensed with, in consequence of the suggestion of my late colleague, Dr Warburton, and myself. *The consequence has been a large diminution in the number of dirty patients ; and by greater attention to the patients before going to bed, the number has been further diminished.*

" Perhaps no example is more striking than the method of treating cases of acute mania in former years, and at the present time. Formerly the patient was strapped down to his bed, and not allowed to move; *the consequence of which was, that the horizontal position favoured the congestion of the brain, and added to the development of the already superabandant nerve-force;* thus producing greater and greater irritation, followed by collapse, typhoid symptoms, and too often by death ; whereas, now, by allowing the patient the free exercise of his limbs, he works off much of the nervous irritation, and by tiring himself out, will *sometimes get to sleep even without a sedative.*"—Ibid., pp. 162, 163.

Walter D. Williams, Esq., M.D., Pembroke House, Hackney.—" In confirmation of which hope, I may

state that the removal of mechanical guards has been
attended with no evil consequences; the pictures and
useful furniture introduced into the day-rooms and
dormitories have met with no injury of any account;
the flowers and fruit have remained in the gardens with
no greater depredation than was intentionally permitted; and the clothing being good and respectable in
appearance, has generally continued to be kept so by
the patients themselves. I may add, that the assem-
bling them together at a common table for their meals,
and allowing them generally the use of knives, so far
from having been followed by any bad result, have,
with the lengthening out of those meals, contributed to
induce habits of quietness, decency, and order. Their
daily country excursions also (in which three-fourths of
their number join), although greatly facilitating the
means of escape, have lessened the inclination to it, and
have tended not only to improve their appearance as to
health and neatness, but also, in conjunction with the
amusements provided for them on their return, to
diminish noisy, restless, and irritable habits; so that, on
the whole, they are thus prepared in some measure for
general society, by occasionally mixing with which their
intellect is roused, their delusions for a time dissipated,
their self-control strengthened, and that hopeless feeling
of exclusion from it at least temporarily removed."—
Ibid., pp. 166, 167.

J. Conolly, Esq., M.D., Hanwell.—" Recollecting
the state of some private Asylums which I visited offi-
cially 30 years ago, I feel perfectly assured that the
amended treatment practised since that period, and

especially the disuse of mechanical restraints of all kinds, has been productive of an incalculable amount of advantage to the insane. The general tranquillity, comfort, and satisfaction visible in all well-conducted Asylums, public and private, attest this in the strongest manner. *Fewer accidents occur; revenge is seldom excited in the minds of the patients; scenes of violence are seldom or never witnessed; the patients manifest no terror; and on recovery, retain no sense of degradation;* often after leaving the Asylum, coming to it again as voluntary visitors to associates and friends, of whose good offices they are fully sensible."—Ibid., p. 171.

E. L. Bryan, Esq., F.R.C.S., Hoxton House.—" With improved premises, increased staff of attendants, and with certain special provisions, I am of opinion that mechanical restraint is not necessary, and that *its disuse is satisfactory and beneficial to the patients."*—Ibid., p. 174.

Alfred G. Kerr, Esq., Grove End Villa, Regent's Park.—" No kind of mechanical restraint is ever resorted to. I have always found that kindness, blended with firmness, *is the most efficient mode of allaying excitement, however violent.* In some cases that have been brought here, the patient has arrived in a strait-waistcoat, on which being removed, *they expressed their thankfulness, and immediately became calm."*—Ibid., p. 175.

R. Langworthy, Esq., Plympton House.—" Mechanical restraint is never had recourse to in this house. I deem it unnecessary where a sufficient number of competent attendants are kept, and the results of the non-restraint system I consider *to have been of great benefit to the insane*."—Ibid., p. 176.

E. V. Henesy, Esq., M.D., High Beech Asylum. — " My experience of the mental treatment is limited; it has, however, been sufficient to force upon me the conviction that mechanical restraint, or over-rigid seclusion, *are the sure means of making maniacs of severe cases, and of greatly aggravating the mildest form of insanity*, by fretting and irritating minds already sufficiently excited."—Ibid., p. 179.

C. Broughton, Esq., Vernon House, Briton Ferry. —" In the treatment of the insane, it is difficult to imagine a case in which mechanical coercion can be deemed advisable, or even allowable. *No instances have fallen under my observation which could seem to justify its employment, or hold out the attainment of any desirable end.*"—Ibid., p. 179.

John George Davey, Esq., M.D., Northwoods, Bristol.—" The time is now gone by when the lunatic was considered within reach only of fear and physical coercion: the more successful means of restraint, as well without as within the Asylum, are derived not from the mere corporeal feelings, but from the brighter side of our common nature; not from fear so much as from love. The gentle remonstrance, when coupled with patience and a kind sympathy, will be more likely to soothe the maniac than anything else. Reply to him in anger, and you aggravate those symptoms of cerebral disorder you would mitigate or relieve."—Ibid., p. 181.

C. H. Newington, Esq., M.D., and S. Newington, Esq., M.D., Ticehurst, Sussex.—" But it is in those patients who have been subjected to mechanical restraint for some time prior to their being removed here, that *the beneficial effeets of withdrawing such restraint have been most especially shown.* Those who, when first admitted, have been mischievous and angry, filthy in their persons and habits, destroying everything fragile they could lay their hands on, thin and haggard in appearance, *have soon become orderly and cleanly, and assumed a marked improvement in their general health and strength,* by being released from their bonds and treated mildly, and as far as possible regarded as rational beings."*—Ibid., p. 200.

W. Berrow, Esq., Duddeston Hall, near Birmingham. —"I have during the last four years been enabled to bear testimony to the great advantages arising from the abolition of mechanical restraint, with a full assurance that such measures *greatly improve the condition, health, and comfort of the insane.*"—Ibid., p. 203.

---

* It is perhaps right to observe that Drs Newington do not advocate the disuse of restraint in all cases.—R. G. H.

ENGLISH ASYLUMS.

ADMISSIONS, PER-CENTAGE OF RECOVERIES, AND DEATHS, FROM 1849 TO 1853.

Description and Number of Asylums.	Admissions.		Recoveries per cent.			Deaths per cent.*		
	M.	F.	M.	F.	M.&F.	M.	F.	M.&F.
County - - - 32	7,937	8,263	33.98	38.78	36.38	10.50	7.39	8 94½
Hospitals (exclusive of Bethlem and St Luke's) - - } 14	1,379	1,270	34.30	38.18	36.24	9.29	6.13	7.71
Licensed Houses - 128	5,886	5,699	34.36	37.21	35.78½	8.44	6.04	7.24
Totals and Average per-centage - - - }	15,202	15,232	34.21	38.05	36.13	9,41	6.52	7.96½

ST LUKE'S HOSPITAL, 1849 TO 1853.

Admissions (Curables).		Recoveries per cent.			Deaths per cent.*		
M.	F.	M.	F.	M.&F.	M.	F.	M.&F.
356	595	55.05	61.34	58.19½	5.65	5.20	5.42½

BETHLEM HOSPITAL, 1852 TO 1856.

Admissions (Curables).		Recoveries per cent.			Deaths per cent.*		
M.	F.	M.	F.	M.&F.	M.	F.	M.&F.
389	652	55.52	60.27	57.89½	5.08	3.10	4.09

* The per centage of deaths is taken upon the numbers under treatment in each year.

COUNTY ASYLUMS, 1854.

ADMISSIONS, NUMBERS UNDER TREATMENT, and per-centage of RE-COVERIES and DEATHS.

Name of Asylum.	Admissions		Number under Treatment.		Recoveries per cent.			Deaths per cent.		
	M.	F.	M.	F.	M.	F.	M. & F.	M.	F.	M. & F.
Bedford - -	32	57	163	200	40.62	33.33	36.97½	6.13	8.	7.06½
Bucks - -	29	19	90	114	31.03	52.63	41.83	11.11	4.38	7.74½
Cheshire - -	52	51	156	192	36.53	39.21	37.87	10.25	7.29	8.77
Cornwall - -	47	49	164	162	31.91	38.77	35.34	11.58	14.19	12.88½
Denbigh - -	44	43	130	143	27.27	41.86	34.56½	9.23	8.39	8.81
Derby - -	76	75	178	166	31.57	33.33	32.45	12.35	6.02	9.18½
Devon - -	53	80	248	329	41.50	37.50	39.50	8.38	8.51	8.44½
Essex - -	204	235	204	235	9.80	13.19	11.48½	23.52	8.51	16.01½
Gloucester -	38	83	196	300	28.94	33.70	31.32	8.67	5.66	7.16½
Hants - -	61	70	169	192	14.75	27.14	20.94½	7.10	7.29	7.19½
Kent - -	97	92	347	402	37.21	41.30	39.25½	14.40	8.45	11.42½
Lancaster -	81	68	416	405	45.67	36.76	41.21½	10.57	9.64	10.10½
Rainhill - -	52	62	243	277	53.84	54.83	54.33½	12.75	7.59	10.17
Prestwich -	119	129	363	360	46.21	51.16	48.68½	17.07	8.88	12.97½
Leicester -	64	67	174	191	28.12	43.28	35.70	8.04	5.23	6.63½
Lincolnshire -	45	25	160	151	40.	56.	48.	11.87	8.60	10.23½
Hanwell - -	87	82	497	640	18.39	17.07	17.73	8.24	6.25	7.24½
Colney Hatch -	254	138	769	867	38.97	31.15	35.06	17.65	8.41	13.03
Monmouth -	44	62	145	195	29.54	37.09	33.31½	13.79	8.20	10.99½
Norfolk - -	34	48	170	211	32.35	56.25	44.30	8.23	6.63	7.43
Oxford - -	67	58	237	282	41.79	41.37	41.58	13.12	6.74	9.93
Salop - -	65	64	186	210	40.	42.18	41.09	8.60	4.76	6.63
Stafford - -	82	83	297	267	45.12	39.75	42.43½	9.76	8.98	9.37
Somerset -	58	65	221	265	44.82	58.46	51.64	13.12	12.45	12.78½
Suffolk - -	34	47	151	191	64.70	51.06	57.88	9.93	7.85	8.89
Surrey - -	161	168	437	663	41.61	44.64	43.12½	13.50	6.63	10.06½
Warwick - -	52	30	138	132	26.92	26.66	26.79	7.97	9.09	8.53
Wilts - -	48	72	158	217	33.33	48.61	40.97	6.32	8.75	7.53½
Worcester -	41	47	143	156	19.51	29.14	24.32½	18.18	16.02	17.10
York, North and East Riding -	36	42	184	189	25.	21.42	23.21	5.43	5.82	5.62½
York, West Riding -	157	171	498	538	41.40	38.59	39.99½	12.24	9.85	11.04½
Totals and average per centage -	2314	2382	7632	8842	35.11	39.27	37.19	11.26	8.16	9.71

COUNTY ASYLUMS, 1855.

ADMISSIONS, NUMBERS UNDER TREATMENT, and per-centage of RECOVERIES and DEATHS.

Name of Asylum.	Admissions		Number under Treatment.		Recoveries per cent.			Deaths per cent.		
	M.	F.	M.	F.	M.	F.	M.&F.	M.	F.	M.&F.
Bedford - -	40	57	178	216	30.	33.33	31.66½	10.11	11.57	10.84
Bucks - -	34	38	104	135	35.29	36.84	36.06½	7.69	4.44	6.06½
Cheshire - -	73	52	181	198	30.13	57.69	43.91	9.39	7.07	8.23
Cornwall - -	41	38	161	154	26.82	39.47	33.14½	8.70	8.44	8.57
Denbigh - -	37	32	133	141	43.24	65.62	54.43	12.03	6.38	9.20½
Derby - -	61	72	183	185	29.50	40.27	34.88½	12.02	3.24	7.63
Devon - -	67	77	204	272	50.74	70.13	60.43½	19.11	5.51	12.31
Dorset - -	23	24	93	107	47.82	45.83	46.82½	7.52	3.73	5.62½
Essex - -	61	68	185	251	36.06	41.17	38.61½	10.81	11.15	10.98
Gloucester -	48	43	191	276	52.08	62.79	57.43½	11.51	5.43	8.47
Hants - -	53	62	198	216	32.07	22.58	27.32½	11.11	7.87	9.49
Kent - -	97	92	347	402	38.14	35.86	37.	14.40	8.45	11.42½
Lancaster -	96	88	424	424	19.79	37.50	28.64½	12.50	6.13	9.31½
Rainhill - -	51	53	230	271	39.21	47.16	43.18½	9.13	7.74	8.43½
Prestwich -	108	106	344	360	39.81	70.75	55.78	10.75	5.83	8.29
Leicester - -	52	53	179	197	34.61	39.43	37.02	8.37	5.07	6.72
Lincolnshire -	32	30	152	153	40.63	33.33	36.98	6.57	8.49	7.53
Hanwell - -	73	78	507	657	24.65	26.92	25.78½	9.86	6.84	8.35
Colney Hatch -	151	59	666	793	27.81	27.11	27.46	13.81	4.53	9.17
Monmouth -	57	43	167	193	49.12	67.44	58.28	14.37	7.77	11.07
Norfolk - -	28	48	165	211	42.85	45.83	44.34	7.27	9.47	8.37
Oxford - -	42	60	216	295	45.23	45.	45.11½	12.08	6.44	9.26
Salop - -	65	43	135	166	44.61	58.13	51.37	12.59	7.83	10.21
Stafford - -	98	76	296	262	41.83	65.78	53.80½	10.13	8.41	9.27
Somerset - -	78	69	241	258	25.64	20.28	22.96	6.22	3.87	5.04½
Suffolk - -	43	40	154	190	23.25	70.	46.62½	11.03	7.89	9.46
Surrey - -	173	133	593	652	41.04	57.89	49.46½	10.79	8.12	9.45½
Warwick - -	42	37	154	145	30.95	32.43	31.69	9.09	11.03	10.06
Wilts - -	69	49	197	210	44.92	55.10	50.01	10.67	10.	10.33½
Worcester -	53	48	157	162	35.84	39.58	37.71	15.28	9.25	12.26½
York., North and East Riding - -	33	34	185	185	27.27	64.70	45.98½	8.64	4.32	6.48
York, West Riding -	134	131	491	529	49.25	62.59	55.92	12.62	6.49	9.55½
Totals and average per-centage -	2113	1933	7811	8876	36.88	47.45	42.16½	10.81	7.15	8.98

COUNTY ASYLUMS, 1856.

ADMISSIONS, NUMBERS UNDER TREATMENT, and per-centage of RE-COVERIES and DEATHS.

Name of Asylum.	Admissions		Number under Treatment.		Recoveries per cent.			Deaths per cent.		
	M.	F.	M.	F.	M.	F.	M. & F.	M.	F.	M. & F.
Bedford - -	57	54	196	214	28.06	48.14	38.10	10.20	11.21	10.70½
Bucks - -	31	33	113	146	35.48	45.45	40.46½	14.15	9.58	11.86½
Cheshire - -	—	—	—	—	—	—	—	—	—	—
Cornwall - -	35	36	156	154	22.85	50.	36.42	15.38	7.79	11.58½
Denbigh - -	38	30	125	136	47.36	50.	48.68	5.60	6.61	6.10½
Derby - -	52	67	187	208	34.61	41.79	38.20	6.41	3.36	4.88½
Devon - -	85	71	200	278	25.88	61.97	43.92½	10.	6.83	8.41½
Dorset - -	26	38	92	120	53.84	44.73	49.28½	4.34	9.16	6.75
Essex - -	70	64	200	259	40.	37.50	38.75	9.56	6.94	8.25
Gloucester - -	51	53	184	268	29.41	32.07	30.74	7.06	5.97	6.51½
Hants - -	83	94	240	273	27.71	38.29	33.	9.58	9.15	9.36½
Kent - -	108	84	355	400	35.18	39.28	37.23	11.26	5.25	8.25½
Lancaster - -	95	91	434	442	23.15	26.37	24.76	11.29	6.10	8.69½
Rainhill - -	42	50	223	268	66.66	66.66	66.66	7.17	5.22	6.19½
Prestwich - -	83	113	333	365	46.98	55.75	51.36½	9.60	7.94	8.77
Leicester - -	57	50	192	210	40.35	60.	50.17½	8.85	5.71	7.28
Lincolnshire -	35	33	162	161	31.42	24.24	27.83	7.40	6.21	6.80½
Hanwell - -	80	60	514	645	31.25	36.66	33.95½	7.21	5.42	6.31½
Colney Hatch -	137	140	651	872	27.73	18.57	23.15	11.67	6.99	9.33
Monmouth -	62	54	176	197	40.32	25.92	33.12	11.36	7.11	9.23½
Norfolk - -	41	44	176	202	48.78	43.18	45.98	10.22	9.40	9.81
Oxford - -	59	60	224	308	32.20	46.66	39.43	9.82	5.84	7.83
Salop - -	52	48	149	166	32.69	41.66	37.17½	12.75	8.43	10.59
Stafford - -	92	80	312	266	53.26	60.	56.63	12.11	7.10	9.60½
Somerset - -	73	60	227	253	41.09	58.33	49.71	7.04	7.90	7.47
Suffolk - -	42	47	167	191	50.	38.29	44.14½	9.58	7.85	8.71½
Surrey - -	151	92	558	607	40.39	40.21	40.30	13.44	5.93	9.68½
Warwick - -	46	48	170	161	39.13	33.33	36.23	11.17	6.23	8.70
Wilts - -	39	61	180	221	43.58	57.37	50.47½	8.88	5.42	7.15
Worcester -	41	39	157	174	29.26	35.89	32.57½	10.82	7.47	9.14½
York, North and East Riding - -	58	37	218	190	18.96	24.35	21.65½	7.33	8.42	7.87½
York, West Riding -	141	155	497	566	39.71	43.22	41.46½	10.06	9.71	9.43½
Totals and average per-centage -	2062	1986	7777	8921	37.33	42.73	40.03	9.76	7.16	8.46

COUNTY ASYLUMS, 1854 TO 1856.

Average Recoveries and Deaths per cent.

Name of Asylum.	Recoveries per cent.				Deaths per cent.			
	1854.	1855.	1856.	Average.	1854.	1855.	1856.	Average
Bedford - -	36.97½	31.66½	38.10	35.58	7.06½	10.84	10.70½	9.53½
Bucks - -	41.83	36.06½	40.46½	39.45¼	7.74½	6.06½	11.86½	8.55¾
Cheshire - -	37.87	43.91	—	40.89	8.77	8.23	—	8.50
Cornwall - -	35.34	33.14½	36.42	34.96¾	12.88½	8.57	11.58½	11.01¼
Denbigh - -	34.56½	54.43	48.68	45,89	8.81	9.20½	6.10½	8.04
Derby - -	32.45	34.88½	38.20	35.17¾	9.18½	7.63	4.88½	7.23¼
Devon - -	39.50	60.43½	43.92½	47.62	8.44½	12.31	8.41½	9.72¼
Dorset - -	—	46.82½	49.28½	48.05½	—	5.62½	6.75	6.18¾
Essex - -	11.48½	38.61½	38.75	29.61½	16.01½	10.98	8.25	11.74¾
Gloucester -	31.32	57.43½	30.74	39.83	7.16½	8.47	6.51½	7.38¼
Hants -	20.94½	27.32½	33.	27.09	7.19½	9.49	9.36½	8.68¼
Kent - -	39.25½	37.	37.23	37.82¾	11.42½	11.42½	8.25½	10.36¾
Lancaster -	41.21½	28.64½	24.76	31.54	10.10½	9.31½	8.69½	9.37
Rainhill - -	54.33½	43.18½	66.66	54.72½	10.17	8.43½	6.19½	8.26½
Prestwich -	48.68½	55.78	51.36½	51.94¼	12.97½	8.29	8.77	10.01
Leicester - -	35.70	37.02	50.17½	40.96½	6.63½	6.72	7.28	6.87¾
Lincolnshire -	48.	36.98	27.83	37.60¼	10.23½	7.53	6.80½	8.19
Hanwell - -	17.73	25.78½	33.95½	25.82¼	7.24½	8.35	6.31½	7.30¼
Colney Hatch -	35.06	27.46	23.15	28.55½	13.03	9.17	9.33	10.51
Monmouth -	33.31½	58.28	33.12	41.57	10.99½	11.07	9.23½	10.43
Norfolk - -	44.30	44.34	45.98	44.87¼	7.43	8.37	9.81	8.53½
Oxford - -	41.58	45.11½	39.43	42.04	9.93	9.26	7.83	9.—½
Salop - -	41.09	51.37	37.17½	43.21	6.63	10.21	10.59	9.14
Stafford - -	42.43½	53.80½	56.63	50.95½	9.37	9.27	9.60½	9.41½
Somerset - -	51.64	22.96	49.71	41.43½	12.78½	5.01½	7.47	8.43
Suffolk - -	57.88	46.62½	44.14½	49.55	8.89	9.46	8.71½	9.02
Surrey - -	43.12½	49.46½	40.30	44.29½	10.06½	9.45½	9.68½	9.73½
Warwick -	26.79	31.69	36.23	31.57	8.53	10.06	8.70	9.06¼
Wilts - -	40.97	50.01	50.47½	47.15	7.53½	10.33½	7.15	8.34
Worcester -	24.32½	37.71	32.57½	31.53½	17.10	12.26½	9.14½	12.83½
York, North and East Riding - -	23.21	45.98½	21.65½	30.28¼	5.62½	6.48	7.87½	6.66
York, West Riding -	39.99½	55.92	41.46½	45.79¼	11.04½	9.55½	9.43½	6.67¾
General average	37.19	42.16½	40.03	39.79½	9.71	8.98	8.46	9.05

SOCIAL CONDITION OF 7,821 PATIENTS UNDER TREAT-
MENT IN COUNTY LUNATIC ASYLUMS.

—	Males.	Females.	Total.	Per centage.		
				M.	F.	M. & F.
Married -	1,752	1,780	3,532	46.51	43.90½	45.20¾
Single -	1,718	1,744	3,462	45.60½	43.02	44.31¼
Widowed -	297	530	827	7.88½	13.07½	10.48
Totals -	3,767	4,054	7,821	100.	100.	100.

TOTAL ABOLITION OF PERSONAL RESTRAINT IN THE
TREATMENT OF THE INSANE.

A

LECTURE

ON

The Management of Lunatic Asylums,

AND THE

TREATMENT OF THE INSANE;

DELIVERED AT THE MECHANICS' INSTITUTION, LINCOLN,
ON THE 21st OF JUNE, 1838:

WITH

STATISTICAL TABLES,

ILLUSTRATIVE OF THE COMPLETE PRACTICABILITY OF THE SYSTEM
ADVOCATED IN THE LECTURE

BY

ROBERT GARDINER HILL,

MEMBER OF THE ROYAL COLLEGE OF SURGEONS, LONDON ;

HOUSE-SURGEON OF THE LINCOLN LUNATIC ASYLUM.

PREFACE.

The object of the following Lecture is simply to advocate the Total Abolition of Severity, of every species and degree, as applied to patients in our Asylums for the Insane; and with this view to shew,—*First*, that such Abolition is in theory highly desirable, and *Secondly*, That it is practicable: in proof of which assertions the present state of the Lincoln Lunatic Asylum is adduced. There such a system is in actual and successful operation—the theory verified by the practice.* It may be proper to state here, that the

---

* The want of information upon this subject, even in respectable quarters, is much to be lamented, and is too well proved by extracts from the Glasgow and Nottingham Reports. Were the matter a theoretical question, such language as theirs might be used: but experience and facts cannot be evaded by mere words. Let our Glasgow and Nottingham neighbours honestly *make the attempt*, and they will succeed: and the necessity for " taking a month to tame a patient " (words lately addressed to me by an attendant at the Glasgow Asylum in excuse for restraining a new patient) will disappear. Such matters should not be left to the discretion of the attendants.

Extract from the Twenty-fifth Annual Report of the Directors of the Glasgow Royal Asylum for Lunatics. 1839.

" In connection with other improvements in the treatment of the insane, we, at an early period of our Institution, made it our especial

principle of Mitigation of Restraint to the utmost extent
that was deemed consistent with safety, was ever the
principle pressed upon the attention of the Boards of
the Lincoln Asylum by its humane and able Physician,
Dr Charlesworth: at his suggestion many of the more
cruel instruments of restraint were long since destroyed,
very many valuable improvements and facilities
gradually adopted, and machinery set in motion, which
has led to the unhoped for result of actual Abolition,
under a firm determination to work out the system to
its utmost applicable limits.   To his steady support,
under many difficulties, I owe chiefly the success which
has attended my plans and labours.   He originated the
requisite alterations and adaptations in the building,

---

study to render the means of coercion, when necessary, as gentle and
as little irritating as possible ; but some degree of personal restraint is
in many cases indispensable, and however gratifying the idea may be to
the speculative philanthropist, the entire abolition of coercion is too
often compensated by concealed severity.   When we hear a vulgar and
uneducated Keeper boasting that, by a glance of his eye, or the turn of
his finger. he can control a whole ward of the Insane, we can guess
pretty well how this seemingly mysterious power was acquired ; and it
would be well if those who visit Mad-houses would carefully study the
countenances of the lunatics when the Keeper approaches, and when he
turns his back to the patient.   An attentive observer might thus sometimes discover a strong and instructive contrast between the subdued
and counterfeited expression in the one case, and the suspicious and
revengeful scowl in the other."

*Extract from the Twenty-eighth Annual Report of the state of the
General Lunatic Asylum, near Nottingham.   1838.*

 " Without entertaining Utopian ideas, on the subject of the total
abolition of all restraint in the treatment of insanity, constant and
unwearied attention has been directed to do as much without it as the
welfare and safety of the insane would admit."

and threw every other facility in the way of accomplishing the object.

Experience has shown that the mere partial mitigation of restraint is not in itself a safe system, suicides not having diminished under it;* if any conclusion may be drawn from the few cases, it would appear on the contrary that there is not any safety, when the attendants are not compelled to rely wholly upon inspection. This propensity cannot be counteracted by any other means than the constant supervision of attendants by day, and a watch by night, aided by the remission of ignorant and cruel usages which no doubt have often driven the insane sufferer to seek in suicide the only means of escape. The disappearance of suicide under the system of Total Abolition has confirmed this opinion. By the annexed Tables it will be seen, that not one fatal accident has occurred in this Asylum since the Total Abolition of Restraints.

The Appendix (A) abounds in curious and instructive matter, which will be found eminently useful in other Institutions. It contains the proceedings of the Boards and Officers for a course of years in carrying out the great principles of Construction, Classification, Public Inspection, Pervision, exoneration of the attendants from domestic duties, and other matters which have directly or indirectly borne upon the final extinction of restraint. These memoranda are peculiarly valuable, as not being merely wild and exaggerated views of the moment, but matters of practice slowly, gradually, and perseveringly worked out from point to

* See Table of Suicides, p. 172.

point, as experience and an indefatigable spirit of benevolence directed the course. The Author is proud to have learned in such a school, and gladly owns the obligation.

LINCOLN LUNATIC ASYLUM,
April 13, 1839.

☞ The Author has not thought it necessary to re-publish the Appendix, or the Statistical Tables accompanying the Lecture, as they are entirely irrelevant to the object of this Historical Sketch, and moreover are easily accessible to any who may wish to consult them, in the Reports of the Lincoln Lunatic Asylum.

A LECTURE,

etc. etc.

Mr President,

    Ladies and Gentlemen,

        In addressing you this evening, I have at least two decided advantages:—In the first place, I need not enter into any lengthened exposition of my design,—I need not explain a mass of difficult and technical phrases, as a necessary preliminary to the right understanding of what I propose to lay before you. Happily my subject requires not such aid: it has *one* recommendation, and that one I believe to be all-sufficient to win your favourable attention:—it asks nothing of you beyond the exercise of your own good sense and benevolent feelings, to make you understand and take an interest in its objects. I plead the cause of a class of your fellow-creatures, too long, alas! neglected, but surely a class demanding, if ever any did demand, the sympathy of every humane heart, and the compassion of every feeling bosom. Such a cause, however little it may derive from its advocate, will never be dismissed hence without an attentive hearing.—In the next place, I have not far to search for an example illustrative of the practice to which I shall this evening direct your

attention. Turn your eyes to that noble Edifice, which
is at once one of the greatest ornaments of modern
date which this City can boast, and a lasting memorial
of your charity and benevolence. Thence are derived
all my materials: there I have not only matured the
plans, but have also witnessed and rejoiced in their
complete success. There at this moment they are in
full operation; and, I may be allowed to state, they
have already produced results beyond even my own
most sanguine expectations. I do not ask your assent
to my unsupported assertion of this: the Tables I have
drawn up, and which I now hold in my hand, are a
proof of it. Thence therefore I derive the illustration
of my theory;—practical results which may be seen and
examined by any of you ;—examples of success which
cannot be gainsayed—which cannot be controverted.
It is no visionary scheme;—the proof is open to all that
I now address.

Counting, therefore, upon a kind and favourable reception from you, I come at once to the point, and ask
whether, after having raised such a noble edifice as the
Lincoln Lunatic Asylum for a class of beings who have
no other hope of recovery on this side the grave, it be
not worth while to consult their personal comfort and
happiness, especially if that comfort and that happiness
be found by experience mainly conducive to their early
restoration to health and sanity, and consequently conducive also in the highest degree to the charitable
objects for which the building was erected? I antici-
pate the answer of every one of you: but readily as this
is granted, conformable as it is to the plain and obvious

dictates of sense and humanity, the history and experience of past times will show us that this principle has not been acted upon in the case of the poor maniac—far from it. The inmates of a Lunatic Asylum (I speak not of our own in particular—its date being comparatively recent, just when a more enlightened system had begun to dawn,—but of every one without exception throughout the whole continent of Europe), were treated more like the savage and untameable beast of the forest than as human beings; and the bare recital of their sufferings under this system of cruelty is almost too horrible to be heard of or to be believed. The testimonies and facts which I shall bring forward will, however, show that I have not overdrawn the picture.

Of the utility, however, of such Institutions, when conducted on humane principles, and when every effort, regardless of trouble or inconvenience, is concentrated towards one grand point—the benefit of the patient—there can be but one opinion. I shall not here dilate on the nature and causes of insanity; although this is a subject which would furnish matter well worthy the consideration, not only of professional men, but also of the philanthropist, the moralist, and even the divine. But it would lead me into a wider field than I have opportunity at present to range through and explore. My only wish, with reference to this part of my subject, is to furnish you with such information as may show you the improbability (I had almost said moral impossibility) of an insane person's regaining the use of his reason, except by removing him early to some Institution for that purpose. If such a result is ever attained without the adoption of this plan, it is either a very rare occurrence indeed, or it has ensued from change of residence, of scene, and of persons around, combined with a mode of treatment in some measure resembling that which can be fully adopted only in a building constructed for the purpose.*

---

* "In any Asylum the patient is more carefully watched, and with less restraint than in a private house. What can be done with a furious individual in an apartment or in a house, however large it might be? For the sake of his own preservation, it would be necessary to tie him down to his bed, which would increase his delirium and fury, while in an Asylum he might indulge in his incoherence with less danger to himself and others. There, too, the management is better understood, the servants are more experienced, and the arrangement of the building allows the patient to be removed from one part to another according to his condition, the efforts which he makes, and his approach to reason."

"Their number (i. e. of the attendants) exhibits an amount of power which overcomes the most furious patient, and very frequently renders the employment of force unnecessary. A patient might be tempted to resist one or two; but when he sees a body of four or five calm, powerful, and determined individuals, ready on the instant to execute the orders of the superintendent, the folly and fruitlessness of any resistance becomes too apparent to allow him to make any effort."

"Example, which has such power over the determinations of men in general, exerts a great influence over the insane. We must bear in mind that the insane frequently exhibit great sagacity in judging of what passes around them. The cure and departure of one patient inspires others with confidence, the hope of recovery, and an assurance that they too will be liberated when cured."

"The care bestowed on them in the bosom of their own families makes no good impression on them, while the attention which they receive from strangers is appreciated from its being new, and their having no right to expect it."—*Edinburgh Medical and Surgical Journal, Jan.* 1. 1839, *pages* 152, 153, *and* 154.

On the first attack of insanity (from whatever cause arising) there is either some one all-engrossing idea haunting the brain like a spectre, and continually suggested so long as the patient remains in the same place, and surrounded by the same persons ;—or there is a strong dislike conceived against the latter, or some one or more of them;—or there is a moping melancholy with an inclination to suicide, which is increased by a continuance among the same objects;—or lastly, there is an unmanageable violence, which vents itself on every thing within its reach, and frequently in attempting to destroy the lives of others: and in all these cases, so long as the patient remains at home, *the exciting causes are continually present and active.* A change of scene is therefore necessary—a change of attendants is necessary—a system of watchfulness is necessary—and many other requisites are necessary, which cannot be even attempted except in an Asylum. A private dwelling is ill adapted to the wants and requirements of such an unfortunate being, as will appear from the sequel of my address; nor is it consistent with the safety of others, that he should be allowed to roam at large. Means are therefore resorted to, which, however indispensable under *such* circumstances, generally complete the misery of the patient, who is thereby cut off, perhaps for ever, from all hope of recovery. And even if a private dwelling did contain all that is requisite, still there is little probability that the patient could derive much benefit from the management of persons, who are neither acquainted with a proper system of treatment, nor, if they were, could they possibly adopt it, and at the same time attend to any other business or occupation whatsoever. *A lunatic demands the whole time and attention of his Guardians.*—In last year's Report of the Lincoln Asylum the following passage occurs: " It cannot be too widely made known that in a properly-constructed and well-regulated Asylum, the insane may be treated not only much more easily and effectually, but also *much more mildly* than at their own homes, where the unadapted arrangements of the dwelling and grounds, and the presence of relatives and dependants, oppose unceasing impediments to recovery, and often produce an aggravation of the complaint by the restraint and close confinement which may become unavoidable under the circumstances."*—Indeed it is not to be expected that a patient should have anything like the same prospect of recovery under improper, as under proper treatment. If it were possible that we could have a return of the number of persons recovering under private† treatment compared with the whole number of lunatics subjected to such treatment, the truth of my observation would be amply verified. Of this, however, we have full proof, that the early removal of patients to a building where proper attendance and care can be had, is essential, *the probability of recovery decreasing in proportion to the length of time which may have elapsed between the period of the attack and that of the removal.* This fact, together with the certain knowledge that a large proportion are yearly

---

* Report for 1837, page 5.

† By private treatment I mean simply treatment at their homes, by their own friends.

discharged reeovered from such Establishments, is sufficiently demonstrative of their utility. " Drs Monro,
Burrows, and Ellis, declare that they cure 90 out of
every 100 cases. Such a result proves, so far as the
practice of these observers is concerned, that Insanity,
instead of being the most intractable, is the most
curable of all diseases. Observe, however, that this
declaration *applies only to recent cases, which have not
existed for more than three months,* and which have
been treated under the most favourable circumstances;
as the patients either belonged to the independent
classes, or were inmates of one of the most deservedly
popular Institutions in England."* But, even taking
the average proportion of cures without reference to
such favourable circumstances, (and this surely is the
safest plan), it ranks very high. In the Lincoln
Asylum the recoveries per 100 patients of every date,
average 38.3;† while the deaths (including not only
deaths from maniacal exhaustion, and from suicide, but
also from old age, from diseases, in short from every
natural cause to which Lunatics, as well as others, are
equally liable) average only 19.5† out of every 100.

---

* Browne on Insanity and Asylums for the Insane, page 69.

† Farr on the Statistics of English Lunatic Asylums, pages 6
and 9.

From the opening of the Institution, April 26, 1820, to December
31, 1838.

Recoveries per cent. (Re-admitted cases included) - 39.86
————————— (Re-admitted cases struck off) - 48.30
Deaths per cent. (Re-admitted cases included) - - 16.50
————————— (Re-admitted cases struck off) - 20.00

R. G. H.

K

At Hanwell, which until very lately was conducted by
Sir William Ellis, the proportion of deaths is somewhat
greater, viz., 50.4* out of every 100. Recoveries
18.8.* It may be observed that Sedentary Employments are encouraged at Hanwell, which has not been
the case at Lincoln.†

The efficacy and utility of asylums being indisputably established, it may be asked, ' How is it to be
accounted for that so strong a feeling should exist against
them, and that so large a majority of patients should be
unwilling to enter them?' The question is natural, and
the answer is easy. If Asylums were now what they
formerly were, little indeed could be urged in their
favour. " There are few subjects into which man can
enquire," says an able Journalist, "from which he will
turn with as much horror, as from an investigation into
the manner in which insane persons were formerly treated.
Lashings, it is recorded, constituted the common mode
of treatment received by these unhappy creatures at the
hands of their ascetical keepers. When Asylums became
general, the case was very little amended. Lunatics
were regarded rather in the light of wild beasts, than

---

* Farr on the Statistics of English Lunatic Asylums, pages 6
and 9.

† I am decidedly opposed to all Employment of Lunatics by which
dangerous implements are put into their hands. It is even proverbial
that

* * * * " edged tools,
Should not be placed in the hands of fools."

More accidents have arisen from this cause, perhaps, than any other.
Besides air and exercise are more suited to such patients, and better
calculated to restore the mind to cheerfulness and sanity.

of human beings, and the mode of managing them corresponded with this brutal and unworthy notion. In fact, neither medical men, nor the public at large, had any hope of a cure of the insane. Their rooms or cells were uniformly loathsome from dirt; and in many places on the Continent, lunatics were confined in cages, through the bars of which food and straw were thrust in to them, and where they were daily exhibited to visitors, who paid a certain sum to see them, as is done with wild beasts."

" This picture might be greatly extended, but enough has been said for our present purpose. And to what period, think you, does this description apply ? It is scarcely 20 years since nearly every word of it might be said with truth of the receptacles of the insane in Britain ! It was only at that period that a better spirit spread abroad on the subject of Insanity. Asylums began to be regarded as places for the cure, not for the living burial, of lunatics."*

I have chosen to give this account in the words of another, that I might not be charged with giving an overdrawn picture; but in truth what has been said is but a mere sketch of their wrongs. Instances could be brought forward, confirmed by undeniable testimony, of brutality at which the mind recoils with horror: but humanity will draw a veil over the unsightly picture, and only express a hope that the system, if not its tragic records, will ere long be buried in oblivion.

Yet while we are compelled to confess that such was

---

* 'Chambers' Edinburgh Journal,' No. 307.

the treatment adopted in cases of insanity, at no very distant period, can we wonder that a feeling, and a very strong feeling too, should be frequently manifested by the afflicted and their friends against entering these retreats? It is only surprising that so much of this feeling has been overcome as is actually the case. The only account that can be given—the only pretext—the only shadow of an excuse that can be alleged in palliation is, that insanity was deemed incurable, and the insane person a dangerous and ferocious animal, who could never again be approached with safety, nor recovered from his savage and destructive habits. The moment this error was exploded, a brighter day began to dawn upon the poor maniac. "Earlier than 20 years ago, a reforming impulse had been given to the subject in some European countries; but the spirit of improvement was tardy in its operation."* It is not my intention to trace fully its rise and progress; but I cannot avoid placing before you a sketch of the first practical attempt at rational and moral treatment; and a more affecting account is not, I think, to be met with in the annals of our race.

"Towards the end of 1792, Pinel, after having many times urged the Government to allow him to unchain the maniacs of the Bicêtre, but in vain, went himself to the authorities, and with much earnestness and warmth, advocated the removal of this monstrous abuse—Couthon, a member of the commune, gave way to M. Pinel's auguments, and agreed to meet him at the

---

* 'Chambers' (ubi supra).

Bicêtre. Couthon then interrogated those who were chained, but the abuse he received, and the confused sounds of cries, vociferations, and clanking of chains in the filthy and damp cells, made him recoil from Pinel's proposition. 'You may do what you will with them, said he, 'but I fear you will become their victim.' Pinel instantly commenced his undertaking. There was about 50 whom he considered might without danger to the others be unchained, and he began by releasing twelve, with the sole precaution of having previously prepared the same number of strong waistcoats, with long sleeves, which could be tied behind the back, if necessary. The first man on whom the experiment was to be tried was an English captain, whose history no one knew, as he had been in chains 40 years. He was thought to be one of the most furious among them; his keepers approached him with caution, as he had in a fit of fury killed one of them on the spot with a blow from his manacles. He was chained more rigorously than any of the others. Pinel entered his cell unattended, and calmly said to him, 'Captain, I will order your chains to be taken off, and give you liberty to walk in the court, if you will promise me to behave well and injure no one.' Yes, I promise you,' said the maniac; 'but you are laughing at me, you are all too much afraid of me.' 'I have six men,' answered Pinel, 'ready to enforce my commands, if necessary. Believe me then on my word, I will give you your liberty if you will put on this waistcoat.'

"He submitted to this willingly, without a word: his chains were removed, and the keepers retired, leaving the door of the cell open. He raised himself many times from his seat, but fell again on it, for he had been in a sitting posture so long that he had lost the use of his legs; in a quarter of an hour he succeeded in maintaining his balance, and with tottering steps came to the door of his dark cell. His first look was at the sky, and he cried out enthusiastically, 'how beautiful!' During the rest of the day he was constantly in motion, walking up and down the staircases, and uttering short exclamations of delight. In the evening he returned of his own accord into his cell, where a better bed than he had been accustomed to had been prepared for him, and he slept tranquilly. During the two succeeding years which he spent in the Bicêtre, he had no return of his previous paroxysms, but ever rendered himself useful by exercising a kind of authority over the insane patients whom he ruled in his own fashion.

" The next unfortunate being whom Pinel visited was a soldier of the French Guards, whose only fault was drunkenness: when once he lost self-command by drink he became quarrelsome and violent, and the more dangerous from his great bodily strength. From his frequent excesses, he had been discharged from his corps, and he had speedily dissipated his scanty means. Disgrace and misery so depressed him that he became insane: in his paroxysms he believed himself a general, and fought those who would not acknowledge his rank. After a furious struggle of this sort, he was brought to the Bicêtre in a state of the greatest excitement. He had now been chained for ten years, and with greater care than the others, from his having frequently broken his chains with his hands only. Once when he broke

loose, he defied all his keepers to enter his cell until
they had each passed under his legs; and he compelled
eight men to obey this strange command. Pinel, in
his previous vists to him, regarded him as a man of
original good nature, but under excitement, incessantly
kept up by cruel treatment; and he had promised
speedily to ameliorate his condition, which promise
alone had made him more calm. Now he announced to
him that he should be chained no longer, 'and to prove
that he had confidence in him, and believed him to be a
man capable of better things, he called upon him to
assist in releasing those others who had not reason like
himself; and promised, if he conducted himself well, to
take him into his own service.' The change was sudden
and complete. No sooner was he liberated than he
became obliging and attentive, following with his eye
every motion of Pinel, and executing his orders with as
much address as promptness: he spoke kindly and
reasonably to the other patients, and during the rest of
his life was entirely devoted to his deliverer. And ' I
can never hear without emotion (says Pinel's son) the
name of this man, who some years after this occurrence
shared with me the games of my childhood, and to
whom I shall feel always attached.'

" In the next cell were three Prussian soldiers, who
had been in chains for many years, but on what account
no one knew. They were in general calm and inoffensive, becoming animated only when conversing together
in their own language, which was unintelligible to
others. They were allowed the only consolation of
which they appeared sensible,—to live together. The

preparations taken to release them alarmed them, as they imagined the keepers were come to inflict new severities; and they opposed them violently when removing their irons. When released they were not willing to leave their prison, and remained in their habitual posture. Either grief or loss of intellect had rendered them indifferent to liberty.

"Near them was seen an old priest, who was possessed with the idea that he was Christ: his appearance indicated the vanity of his belief; he was grave and solemn; his smile soft and at the same time severe, repelling all familiarity; his hair was long and hung on each side of his face, which was pale, intelligent, and resigned. On his being once taunted with a question that 'if he was Christ he could break his chains,' he solemnly replied, 'Frustra tentaris Dominum tuum.' His whole life was a romance of religious excitement. He undertook on foot pilgrimages to Cologne and Rome, and made a voyage to America for the purpose of converting the Indians: his dominant idea became changed into actual mania, and on his return to France he announced himself as the Saviour. He was taken by the Police before the Archbishop of Paris, by whose orders he was confined in the Bicêtre as either impious or insane. His hands and feet were loaded with heavy chains, and during twelve years he bore with exemplary patience this martyrdom and constant sarcasms. Pinel did not attempt to reason with him, but ordered him to be unchained in silence, directing at the same time that every one should imitate the old man's reserve, and never speak to him. This order was rigorously observed, and produced on the patient a more decided effect than either chains or a dungeon; he became humiliated by this unusual isolation, and after hesitating for a long time, gradually introduced himself to the society of the other patients. From this time his notions became more just and sensible, and in less than a year he acknowledged the absurdity of his previous prepossession, and was dismissed from the Bicêtre.

"In the course of a few days, Pinel released fifty-three maniacs from their chains: among them were men of all conditions and countries; workmen, merchants, soldiers, lawyers, &c. The result was beyond his hopes. Tranquillity and harmony succeeded to tumult and disorder, and the whole discipline was marked with a regularity and kindness which had the most favourable effect on the insane themselves; rendering even the most furious more tractable."*

Previous to this trial moral and humane treatment was never attempted. "The mind was left to recover its native strength and buoyancy spontaneously."† "Classification was never thought of: criminals, lunatics, the furious and the gentle, were compelled to live promiscuously."‡ Instruments of restraint of the most cruel description were constantly resorted to; instruments which deprived the patient of all power and command over himself, and reduced him at once to the most abject state of helplessness, misery, filth, and

---

* The British and Foreign Medical Review, No. 1, page 286.
† Browne on Insanity and Asylums for the Insane, page 223.
‡ Ibid.

wretchedness. Food was thrust down the throat, and the mouth forced open by one of those instruments of cruelty, the use of which was occasionally attended with fatal results. The wretched victims of this barbarous system were left to wallow in their filth on heaps of straw—no fires allowed—their extremities sometimes in a state of mortification through excessive cold—and not even the sexes separated from each other.

I turn with pleasure from this picture to the more humane and more enlightened system which followed the attempt of the intelligent and immortal Pinel, and in which the Quakers took the lead in this country in their admirable Institution the Retreat. To the credit of all concerned, it may be truly asserted, that when once it was proved that moral means were efficacious, improvement rapidly advanced. Everywhere the light seemed to flash upon mankind, that these unfortunate beings were still of the same race and order with themselves, and had some claim to an attempt at least at kind and feeling treatment. The attempt once made, its efficacy was undeniable; and now there does not exist an Institution where *kindness* is not held forth as the principal means resorted to for the recovery of the insane. The very name of "Mad-house" is almost forgotten. In place thereof an "Asylum" is offered for these poor creatures:—a place of refuge, of shelter from injury, of comfortable retreat, until the storm be over-past:—a place where every want is attended to, every reasonable wish gratified. Still, however, much remains to be done: and it is mainly with the view of stating what may yet be accomplished, and not merely stating, but proving that statement by incontestible examples. that I now address you. I wish to complete that which Pinel began. I assert then in plain and distinct terms, that in a properly-constructed building, with a sufficient number of suitable attendants, restraint is never necessary, never justifiable, and always injurious, in all cases of lunacy whatever. I assert the possibility of the total banishment of instruments of restraint, and all other cruelties whatsoever. I assert that the Asylum of your own City, when completed, may be conducted without a single instance of restraint occurring from one year's end to another. I trust I may here calculate upon your indulgence when I venture to read an extract or two from the Reports of our Asylum for 1837 and 1838, although they have reference to myself, and my opinions.

(1837.) " The present House-Surgeon has expressed his own belief, founded on experience in this house, that it may be possible to conduct an Institution for the Insane without having recourse to the employment of any instruments of restraint whatsoever. He has certainly made a striking advance towards verifying this opinion, by conducting the male (the completed) side of the house, with but a solitary* instance of such restraint, either by day or by night, during the course of the sixteen last months, and that applied only for

---

* This is an error, there was another instance amounting to eight hours. This occurred in consequence of a bench ordered many months before not having been fixed in the floor, in place of loose forms applicable as instruments of offence by the Patients.

about six hours, during his absence; nor is it impossible, when the buildings can be finished, that an example may be offered of an Asylum, in which undivided personal attention towards the patients shall be altogether substituted for the use of instruments.

" By the degree of approach to this result of sound construction, of management, and of official conduct, ought the excellence of every public Asylum to be tested."*

(1838.) " There is now an increased confidence that the anticipations of the last year may be fulfilled, and that 'An example may be offered of a public Asylum, in which undivided personal attention towards the patients shall be altogether substituted for the use of instruments of restraint.' The bold conception of pushing the mitigation of restraint to the extent of actually and formally abolishing the practice, mentioned in the last Report as due to Mr Hill the House-Surgeon, seems to be justified by the following abstract of a statistical Table, showing the rapid advance of the abatement of restraints in this Asylum, under an improved construction of the building, night-watching, and attentive supervision. We may venture to affirm that this is the first frank statement of the common practice of restraints, hitherto laid before the British Public."† (See the following Table.)

---

* Report for 1837, page 5. † Report for 1838, page 4.

Year.	Total number of Patients in the House	Total number of Patients Restrained.	Total number of instances of Restraint.	Total number of Hours passed under Restraint.
1829*	72	39	1727	20,424
1830	92	54	2364	27,113¾
1831	70	40	1004	10,830
1832	81	55	1401	15,671½
1833	87	44	1109	12,003½
1834	109	45	647	6,597
1835	108	28	323	2,874
1836	115	12	39	334
1837	130	2	3	28

After deducting the number of Patients introduced in the above Table more than once in the years 1829-30-31-32-33-34-35, and also the re-admitted cases within the same period, the actual number of patients restrained in the course of such seven years was, 169 :—

Of these 169, there remained in the house at the end of such seven years, 43 : —

Of these remaining 43, there were discharged from the books during the years 1836-7, *not having been restrained at all* during any part of such two years . 11

————————— having been restrained only for about *seven hours* during any part of such two years . . . .

—————remained in the house December 31,1837, *not having been restrained at all* during any part of such two years - 29

————————— having been restrained *once only* (for about nine hours) during any part of such two years 1

————

43

Suffer me now to bring forward a few examples illustrative of the efficacy of proper treatment without restraint; premising that the very restoration to liberty of patients brought to us under all manner of restraints, and apparently ungovernably furious, has often an immediate good effect in restoring them to repose, and in one or two instances, almost to sanity. Indeed the violence is much oftener the result of coercion than of the malady.

Nos. 547, 549, and 551 :—These patients were ad-

* From March 16th.

mitted in January, 1836. They had all been confined in a workhouse for a number of years—say between fifteen and twenty. During this period of time they scarcely knew what it was to be at liberty; I have understood that they were chained both day and night to their bedsteads, and kept in a state so filthy that it was heart-sickening to go near them. They were usually restrained with the strait-waistcoat, with collars round their necks ;—the collars being fastened with chains or straps to the upper portions of their bedsteads, to prevent them (as I have since been informed) from biting their bed-clothes: their feet were chained to the bedsteads with iron leg-locks, to which chains were attached. One of the poor creatures, who no doubt had her lower extremities at liberty, was so deformed from the continued confinement, that she was unable to move about; her limbs having become contracted to such a degree that her feet were drawn up until the soles were even with the lower part of her back: when moved from one room to another it was necessary for an attendant to carry her. These individuals *have never been personally restrained since their admission:* one of them I once placed under seclusion for a few hours only ; but beyond that, no coercive means whatever have been employed. Two of these patients have been restored to habits of cleanliness :—one in particular now spends the greater part of her time in knitting, sewing, &c. Of course they have not been so orderly in their conduct as many of their companions; but is this to be wondered at, when for such a number of years they had been treated more like brutes than human beings ? The crippled patient died a few months since of consumption.

(1838) April 12.—No. 662, æt. 20.—This patient has been readmitted this afternoon. She was brought in a strait-waistcoat, in a state of the greatest excitement. Five persons could scarcely bring her. She is single, and a member of the Baptist persuasion. This attack came on about a week since; the former about three years ago, from which she recovered after remaining in this Establishment about three or four months. She raves chiefly on religious topics, and is subject to sudden and violent fits of phrenzy. During the former attack she attempted self-destruction by jumping into a stone pit; she occasionally destroys her wearing-apparel. Grief and religious excitement are assigned as the immediate exciting causes of the attack. 8. P.M.—She has been very active in her personal exertions, and is unable to control herself.

April 13.—She has been under watch, and has been restless the whole of the night; she is still very active in her personal exertions, but more tractable than she was yesterday.

April 14.—She has become quiet and orderly.

April 15.—She continues calm and well-behaved.

April 18.—The patient who was brought here on the 12th instant, confined with a strait-waistcoat, and guarded by several attendants, is already so far recovered as to have lost all disposition towards any inordinate action, and has been removed this morning to the Moderate Patients' Gallery. It cannot be doubted, indeed she has herself stated, that *the irritation of per-*

sonal restraint had occasioned the excitement she at first exhibited. The strait-waistcoat was instantly taken off on her admission.

April 20.—She has been removed to the Convalescent Patients' Apartment, and is now employed in needle-work.

From April 20 to June 11 inclusive.—Employed in household-work, needle-work, &c. &c.

June 11.—She has been discharged this day by the Weekly Board of Governors. When discharged she applied for the situation of kitchen-maid, and was engaged.

(1838) April 5.—No. 661, æt. 52.—This man has been received this morning. He is a labourer, married —with a family of six children. He has attended the Church regularly, and has also for many years attended the Wesleyan meetings. The first attack of Insanity he experienced was in his 29th year, when he was confined for thirteen weeks in Mr ——'s Establishment at ——, where he recovered. This his second attack exhibited itself about ten days since, and no cause can be assigned for it except some recent religious excitement. He is subject to sudden fits of phrenzy, in one of which he escaped from his friends in a state of nudity;—he has conceived a strong dislike to the persons who have taken an active part in restraining him. He has neither attempted to injure himself, nor any other person. He has been confined in a strait-waistcoat since the commencement of the attack. Three men accompanied him hither. 8 P.M.—Since his admission he has been rolling about the floor of the Refractory

Patients' Gallery: he has also been jumping and running to and fro';—he has just run violently against the gallery door, and broken it.

April 6.—He is very restless and incoherent, and has been so the whole of the night;—he is again rolling on the floor of the gallery—I have desired the attendant not to leave him, for fear he should get hurt by any of the other patients.

April 7.—Though not so active in his personal exertions he is still restless,—complains of thirst;—I have ordered the attendant to offer him cold water frequently during the day and night. He has slept under watch since his admission.

April 10.—He is not so restless, and is certainly improved in health.

April 14.—He continues to improve.

April 18.—He has lost all disposition to any inordinate action, and has this morning been removed to the Moderate Patients' Gallery.

April 21.—He is rational, quiet, and well-behaved.

April 28.—He has been employed in household work and in gardening, since the 18th instant.

From April 29 to June 11 inclusive.—Has been employed in the wash-house;—has occasionally been allowed to go into the town accompanied by an attendant.

June 11.—Has been discharged this day. (Recovered.)

(1838) April 23.—No. 664, æt. 28.—This patient has been received this morning. He is married, is a labourer, and a member of the Methodist persuasion. He has always been considered a sober, industrious, and respectable person. This his first attack came on a few weeks since, previous to which for a fortnight or three weeks he was observed to be more than usually devout and enthusiastic in his religious exercises. He is subject to sudden fits of phrenzy, but his certificate does not state whether he is dangerous or otherwise. Religious excitement is assigned as the immediate exciting cause of his insanity. It appears the malady has been much aggravated by the use of the strait-waistcoat and other instruments of restraint. The persons accompanying him informed me, that he had been bound down to his bedstead for the three or four last weeks, and that his health was much injured in consequence. His appearance is indeed ghastly, and owing to his long confinement he has not the proper use of his lower extremities. He has also large sores upon his back. 7 P.M.—He has been very quiet since his admission, but is now restless, talkative, and noisy.

April 24.—He has been under watch;—has passed a restless night;—is somewhat noisy this morning, and talks much on religious subjects, fancying that he has converted to his own views the workmen employed at the — Union.

April 25.—He is now tractable.

April 26.—He is improving.

April 30.—He is quiet and orderly, and has been removed to the Moderate Patients' Gallery.

May 1.—He is rational, calm, and well-behaved and has been removed to the Convalescent Patients'

Apartment. He is gaining strength rapidly, and recovering the proper use of his lower extremities.

From May 1 to May 25 inclusive.—Improving in health.

May 26.—He has recovered his health. He has been permitted this day to go beyond the walls, accompanied by an attendant and one of the other patients.

From May 26 to June 11 inclusive.—Employed in the garden, yards, &c.

June 11.—He has been discharged this day. (Recovered.)

This man must have died had the restraint been continued, so much had his health suffered from the impossibility of attending to himself, and to his natural wants.

No. 449.—Farmer. Married man. This furious patient was admitted on the 9th of January, 1834, aged 50. The malady in this case is hereditary, affording a lamentable exemplification of that law of nature —the impress of Nature's God—by which parents transmit to their offspring not merely the outward resemblance of feature, nor the yet more striking individual peculiarities of gait, manner, and action, so often observed to descend in this way;* but also the physical

* Thus far the observation holds good throughout almost the whole animal kingdom, except in cases of transformations, as of the caterpillar to the butterfly ; and it forms that bond of similarity in the same species amid the interminable variety of the individuals that compose it, which is one of the great charms of animated nature.

conformation and constitution of those exquisitely-formed internal organs, so intimately connected with the nobler powers of man—the mind and its energies and operations. Mania, then, being in some instances hereditary, it is clear that in those instances it must depend on some organic conformation or constitution, which is transmitted from sire to son; and from the accurate investigations and experiments made of late years, little doubt remains that the brain is the organ in question. *How*, indeed, a certain conformation of brain is connected with certain mental capacities or mental delusions, or how certain modes of life and conduct conduce to bring about that state of brain in those hereditarily predisposed to it, and even in others not so inheriting that predisposition, remains a subject of curious and not unprofitable speculation. But to return to my narrative. His malady first showed itself in January, 1831. He had then been long given to habits of intoxication, indulging freely in the use of ale and ardent spirits. Foreseeing clearly the effect of these habits, as respected his fortune and means of livelihood, he had a terrible dread of impending poverty; and so horribly did this prospect haunt his imagination, that unable to discontinue those pernicious habits, the dire effects of which he so keenly and remorsefully anticipated, he attempted self destruction by knocking his head violently against a wall. He was, however, discharged on trial on the 24th of October, 1834, having been an inmate of the Asylum nine months and a fortnight. Until the month of June following no symptoms of his former malady appeared, and in that interval he managed his affairs with considerable discretion, and conducted himself with decency, industry, and sobriety. But about the period mentioned he again indulged, as before, in the too free use of fermented liquors, and the consequence was a recurrence of his malady, and he was once more remanded to the Asylum. His friends stated that he had become quite violent and unmanageable, that he had attempted to destroy his wife with a garden-fork, which he had latterly kept in his bed-room, together with a gun and other formidable weapons. They further stated that he had broken some windows at the Rectory of the village where he resided, and that his conduct and demeanour towards several of his neighbours had been violent in the extreme. At the time of my appointment to the Asylum, he was suffering extremely from depression of spirits: he would often weep bitterly, supposing that his soul was for ever lost, and that he was doomed to suffer in hell fire. In the month of August (1835), so bent did he appear on self destruction, that I deemed it necessary to confine him to his bedstead for four successive nights; since which time, although frequently under the influence of violent paroxysms of phrenzy, he has not been personally restrained at all, the Dormitory and Nightwatch (both of which were incipiently brought into operation within a week of the period named) having superseded the use of manacles at night. In May, 1836, being suddenly seized with one of his most outrageous paroxysms, he broke several panes of glass in the Moderate Patients' Apartment, where he had previously to that time conducted himself in a quiet and well-behaved way. In doing this, he cut both his hands and wrists, and wounded one or two blood-vessels: his wounds having been dressed, he was removed without loss of time to the Refractory Patients' Gallery, where he has remained ever since in a state of great mental excitement, occasionally uttering the most profane and impious expressions, blaspheming God, throwing himself into attitudes of defiance, and threatening all around him with immediate and dire revenge. During these paroxysms he is watched most closely by the attendants, who however do not attempt to interfere with him, having found by long experience that even a word in remonstrance is but adding fuel to the fire. He is loud and vociferous, and will stand for hours together shouting to the walls, to the trees, and to the sky, believing that while so engaged he is building castles, palaces, and churches. He was employed for a length of time in his lucid intervals in gardening, trenching, removing soil, &c., but so uncertain was his conduct and demeanour, that it was ultimately considered necessary to keep him altogether unemployed, and to watch him closely. Yet even with this man, no coercive means are used—a proof at once that they may so far be dispensed with. He is believed to be of a cowardly disposition, and is so considered by the attendants. In one of his lucid intervals he informed me that when breaking the windows here, he made no doubt he was at his own village " playing away at the Rectory windows as on a former occasion :" and at the same time he expressed his contrition for having committed such an error. This individual is of athletic form, stands about six feet two inches high, and is of a morose and savage temper, although exhibiting frequently such strong marks of cowardice—but cruelty and cowardice are often strangely blended;—from his youth upwards he has ever been hasty, irritable, and vindictive.*

I beg leave now to read a letter from a patient to her friends :—

"LINCOLN, JANUARY 4, 1837,

" Mrs ——,

"When I was at —— I heard them say I was to come to Lincoln Lunatic Asylum, when I was quite feared seeing the severe confinements ;—but this is quite different :—I am in the wards up and down where there are thirty-three female patients. I have not seen a strait-waistcoat, nor yet leather-sleeves, nor leg-locks, nor muzzles,* or other sorts of confinements ;—say or do what you will there is no fault found;—the nurses all seem very loving and dutiful to the patients. If your finger only aches the House-Surgeon attends several times a day ; and at night if he see any of them unruly he orders a nurse to sit up with them. The bed-rooms are carpeted (feather beds most of them with hangings), wash-stands, basins, towels, looking-glass,

---

* This case was not read for fear of extending the lectures to too great a length. It was written a considerable time previous to the lecture, but as the case is a strong one I have thought proper to insert it.

† Muzzles and even gags have been employed in some Institutions to stifle the noise made by the more violent patients.

comb, and brush, and a nurse to attend us. We have tea twice a day, and as much toast as we can eat;— milk and bread for our supper, meat dinners every day, and different sorts of puddings: the Matron of the Asylum stands at the table, and asks whether we are all satisfied ; and if any one wants more she orders a nurse to bring it:— she wishes to see us all comfortable. We go to bed at eight o'clock ;—we have nothing to do only to walk in the gardens twice a day, and cards to play, and other sorts of exercise. I never was better off since I left my parents."

This proves that the system adopted is gratifying to the patients, and thereby conduces to the comfort and healing of their minds :—it will be necessary to add, that the above patient had been confined in other Institutions for persons in her unfortunate situation.

But, it may be demanded, 'What mode of treatment do you adopt, in place of restraint? How do you guard against accidents? How do you provide for the safety of the attendants' ? In short, what is the substitute for coercion'? The answer may be summed up in a few words. viz, :—

CLASSIFICATION AND WATCHFULNESS.

VIGILANT AND UNCEASING ATTENDANCE BY DAY AND BY NIGHT.

KINDNESS, OCCUPATION, AND ATTENTION TO HEALTH, CLEANLINESS, AND COMFORT; AND

THE TOTAL ABSENCE OF EVERY DESCRIPTION OF OTHER OCCUPATION OF THE ATTENDANTS.

This treatment, in a properly-constructed and suitable building, with a sufficient number of strong and active attendants always at their post, is best calculated to restore the patient; and all instruments of coercion and torture are rendered absolutely and in every case unnecessary.

In order, however, that this plan may be undeviatingly pursued, several essential requisites must unite:—

1. A suitable building must be provided, in an airy and open situation, with ground sufficient for several court-yards, gardens, and pleasure-grounds, commanding (if possible) a pleasing and extensive prospect.

2. There must be a proper classification of the patients, more *especially by night.**

3. There must be also a sufficient number of strong, tall, and active attendants, whose remuneration must be such as to secure persons of good character, and steady principle, to undertake their arduous duties. And

4. The House-Surgeon must exercise an unremitting control and inspection, in order that the plan may never, under any circumstances whatever, be deviated from in the slightest degree.

1 & 2. The nature of the building required will be best understood from a view of the classification, which renders a proper number of Apartments, Dormitories, Galleries, and Court-yards, unavoidably necessary. The following is a view of the classification adopted in our Asylum.

---

* Suicide under this system must be obviated by the constant attention of the House-Surgeon to the proper Classification of the Patients *by night*. Those disposed to suicide should always be placed in an Open Dormitory under watch. *Nothing else can prevent Suicide under any system whatever.*

Degrees of Rank—Three, according to the payments made; viz., First, Second, Third.

Classes of Insanity—Three;—viz., Convalescent and Orderly, Moderate, Disorderly.

The Day apartments consist of fourteen sitting-rooms, six galleries, and six dining-rooms.

The Convalescent and Orderly, and the Moderate of the first Rank have front rooms in the centre part of the House.

The Convalescent and Orderly of the second and third Ranks have front rooms at the extremities of the east and west Wings.

The Moderate patients of the second and third Ranks have the use of Galleries and Sitting-rooms, in the front, on the ground and first floors;—these Galleries and Sitting-rooms have a southern aspect.

The Disorderly of the Three Ranks have the use of Galleries and Sitting-rooms which project northward from the back of the Wings, and have eastern and western aspects respectively.

The patients of the Three Ranks have at all times access to the Courts, and the Convalescent and Orderly, and the Moderate are allowed for many hours during the day to take exercise on the lawn in front of the Establishment. As an indulgence, the quieter patients are allowed occasionally to accompany the porter and attendants into the town;—*i. e.* one or two at a time:—occasionally as many as six females have gone out together into the fields.

The night apartments consist of two Open Galleries or Dormitories, containing eighteen beds each;—two

Watch rooms adjoining the Dormitories, with eight beds each;—also four rooms, with two beds each;—four rooms, with three beds each;—and forty-eight rooms, with one bed each:—besides the above there are two Infirmaries for the first and second rank patients, each containing three beds.

The long Dormitories are used for the patients disposed to self-destruction:—the beds in the Watch-rooms to those who destroy bed-clothing,* and to the epilep-

---

* I cannot forbear giving a case of this description, one of the worst which has come under my observation; in which, nevertheless, the necessity for restraint was obviated by management.

(1838) January 19.—No. 648, æt. 50.—This woman has been received to-day. She has two children. The attack commenced about seven months since: she raves indifferently on various topics; is subject to sudden and violent fits of phrenzy, and is very prone to destroy property. The immediate exciting cause was the loss of her husband who died insane. The patient attended upon him during his illness, and up to his death, when she herself became insane. She is very violent, and has been confined in a strait-waistcoat since the commencement of the attack. She is insensible to the ordinary calls of nature.

January 20.—She has passed a restless night. Her blankets were enclosed in a strong case. She is very active in her personal exertions, and is noisy and unruly.

January 22.—She is very refractory and quarrelsome.

January 25.—She is noisy and refractory.

January 26.—She continues noisy and refractory.

January 27.—She continues inattentive to the ordinary calls of nature. She has destroyed her pillow-case and night-gown. Her blankets are enclosed in a strong case.

January 29.—She tears her clothes, and commits other acts of gross extravagance. A strong dress has been purchased for her.

January 30.—She continues to indulge her destructive propensity. I have desired a nurse to sit by her in the day-time.

February 9.—She has by some means effected an opening into her

tics ;--the rooms containing two and three beds each, to the harmless and convalescent, and the single-bedded

---

blanket-case, and destroyed its contents to the amount of four blankets. I have ordered that the pieces be collected, and quilted within the case.

February 10.—Much quieter during the night than she has been for some time past. The nurse is obliged to remain with her in the day-time, or else she would not only destroy her own clothes, but those belonging to the other patients also.

February 11.—She has been very restless during the night. I have desired the attendant on watch to visit her occasionally, which can be done without neglecting the other patients, by having another nurse to sleep in the watch-room, and both to watch alternately.

February 25.—She is very violent and abusive.

March 8.—She is very incoherent and disorderly.

April 9.—She still continues inattentive to the ordinary calls of nature and shows a strong inclination to destroy property.

April 19.—Having contrived several times of late to destroy her blanket-case, a new case has been provided expressly for her : through this she has made a hole with her teeth of the size of a crown-piece, and has withdrawn the whole of the woollen rags which the case contained. I have therefore ordered that she be removed to the Watch-room, and every natural want regularly and strictly attended to. The result is she has been quiet during the whole of the night, as well as attentive to the requirements of nature.

April 20.—She has been under watch during the night, and I am happy to say has not forfeited herself as regards either her propensity to destroy clothing, or her inattention to the ordinary calls of nature. This individual had been confined in a strait-waistcoat for many months previous to her admission here.

April 26.—She continues attentive to the ordinary calls of nature being under watch. She has certainly the power to control herself, and has latterly endeavoured to do so in the day-time as well as during the night. Previous to her removal to the watch-room, she was told that if she would be cleanly in her habits, she should be treated like the other patients ; that is, instead of having straw to sleep upon, she should have a flock bed. She promised to be clean, and she has certainly kept her word up to the present period.

May 1.—She continues true to her word; and in the day-time,

rooms to the harmless, the noisy, the violent, or the insensible.*

The greatest attention to personal cleanliness is observed. The patients have the use of the warm bath on admission: afterwards once in three weeks, and oftener if necessary: their feet are washed and their heads dry-cleaned once a week, and their hands and faces daily:—their body-linen is changed twice a week; —their bed-linen once in three weeks.

They have always water accessible in the galleries and sitting-rooms, so that it is scarcely possible for them to suffer from thirst.

The house is well ventilated;—the bed-room windows are thrown open immediately after rising, and kept open throughout the day. The gallery and sitting-room windows are opened at meals and when they are taking exercise. They are also kept open during the

---

though she is very incoherent and mischievous, yet she is far more orderly than she used to be.

May 7.—Clean and orderly.

(1839) February 14.—She has continued so ever since. Had this patient been put under restraint, she might have continued for ever a loathsome object, insensible to every natural call : for the case was and is incurable.

* Recent observation has convinced me that if Dormitories could be provided for the Insensible patients also (those, I mean, who do not attend to the calls of nature), with Night-watches, such might speedily be restored to habits of cleanliness. This plan has been attended with the happiest effect in some late instances : and indeed we have now few patients who are dirty in the day-time, why then in the night? Simply because they can be attended to only in the day-time, and if this attendance could be given also in the night, cleanliness and self-control would speedily supervene.

whole of the night. The beds are thrown open, and not made up until breakfast is over.

It may be proper to add, that the apartments are now warmed by open fires,* by which any unwholesome tendency (as well as the expense), of heated air-flues, is avoided. The introduction of sash doors is another excellent feature of this Institution; for which, with his other valuable improvements, too great thanks cannot be given to Dr Charlesworth, our senior physi‑cian. Some expedient is still required for the separa‑tion of the noisy from the quiet at night. I have long seen the necessity of this at Lincoln : these individuals must do considerable mischief to the others, and impede their return to a state of sanity.

3. A sufficient number of tall, strong, and active attendants, is absolutely necessary. The system of watchfulness is one which cannot be dispensed with. They must not be employed in any other way—their whole time and attention must be occupied with their charge. They must not be frequently changed—a change should never be made without actual necessity. They must be well remunerated, in order to secure per‑sons of character and of trust. They must not speak angrily to the patients; nevertheless they must be firm and determined in their demeanour towards them. An attendant ought on no occasion to have more than twelve or fifteen patients under his care. The same

---

* The fire-places, however, are protected by a strong iron guard, lined with fine wire-work, which prevents the introduction of a stick or other combustible by the patients.

number of violent patients will require at least two to observe them. The laws of France assign one keeper to every ten patients.

Neither the patients nor attendants should be supplied with fermented liquors : such allowances have been found to engender strifes and contests amongst the former, and with the latter habits of intemperance, materially affecting the good order of the Establishment. In special cases where stimulants may be required, the faculty have power to order them.

In the treatment of the insane, medicine is of little avail,* except (of course) when they are suffering also from other diseases, to which lunatics as well as sane persons are liable. MORAL TREATMENT WITH A VIEW TO INDUCE HABITS OF SELF-CONTROL, IS ALL AND EVERY-THING. I have spoken of classification and watchfulness : but these things are done by their guardians, and have little or no reference to their feelings ; for they should if possible be watched without leading them to suppose that they are suspected of anything improper or injurious.† But occupation and kindness have especial reference to the patient ; and their object is (as I have

---

* The use of the lancet, leeches, cupping-glasses, blisters, drastic purgatives, and the practice of shaving the head are totally proscribed in this Asylum as at Gloucester. The patients' bowels are kept open, their general health is attended to, and they are allowed a generous diet, but no fermented. liquor. The daily allowance of meat, bread, milk, &c., will be seen on reference to the Diet Table which is appended to this lecture.

† It is essential, however, that the patient should be aware that he is *observed* though not *suspected of wrong:* and aware also that the person who observes him is powerful enough to control him.

stated) to induce habits of self-control and cleanliness, which qualities are both essential to recovery, and yet cannot possibly be attained unto by a patient under restraint. Out-door employments with moderate exercise—cheerful society—the occasional presence of friends and even of visitors—healthy recreations and amusements—the enjoyment of the sweet music of spring, of a calm summer evening—the care of a garden or a shrubbery, or the cultivation of rare and choice flowers—all unite in producing a healthy tone, and giving nerve and vigour to the shattered mind. No patient should be COMPELLED to work in any way; but many of them, both males and females, will voluntarily make themselves useful and be industrious ; and in many cases their services are very valuable. Sedentary employments are not good. The offices of religion have a soothing and favourable effect on many :—I have found the use of evening service, and the calm and sober strain of piety which pervades the Liturgy, to be well adapted to these unfortunate beings. Religious excitement of the feelings is always bad, and has brought a great number of patients to this, as well as to every other Asylum. A patient should never be terrified. "Fear is known, by those who have studied the feelings under which self-destruction is attempted, to be one of its most frequent causes. Strange to say, the apprehension of death itself leads to this act. 'It would seem,' says Dr Reid, 'as if they rushed into the arms of death in order to shield themselves from the terror of his countenance.'"*

* Browne on Insanity and Asylums for the Insane, page 29.

Their feelings should be consulted as far as possible :—
the bath of surprise, the rotatory chair, and all such
devices cannot have a good effect.

Undivided personal attention towards the patients
is now altogether substituted in this Establishment for
the use of Instruments. During the last year there
were but three instances of Restraint, and those amongst
the females; arising entirely from the unfinished and
crowded state of the House, as did the two on the male
side during the preceding year. When appointed House-
Surgeon I confess I was but inexperienced; for on finding patients under restraint I kept them so, merely
because the attendants wished me so to do. Had their
wishes alone been consulted, no doubt such treatment
would have continued to the present time; but I soon
observed that the wish on their part was a mere pretext
for idleness, and a short time subsequent to this, I refused altogether to comply with their requests. Matters
went on pretty well for three months; when the calls for
restraint appeared so urgent, that I was induced to give
way, and again the inmates were treated on the old
principle. This was kept up for a few weeks, during
which time I bestowed much attention on the patients,
and observed frequently and assiduously the conduct of
the attendants towards them. At length I felt convinced
there was little occasion for the restraint, and resolved
within myself to discontinue its use altogether. With
this determination, I set at liberty those that were
actually coerced; and from that time to the present,
have had no occasion to resort to such measures, except
in a few instances which arose, as I have before stated,

M

from the unfinished and too crowded state of the Establishment. For a while after this I was frequently applied to for restraint, but on each occasion I have refused it on the ground that it was unnecessary, having first visited the patient, and enquired into the circumstances. Thus it appears, that unless a Superintendent himself actually inspects the whole, and sees that his directions are accurately observed, he may be imposed upon, and the patients exposed to unnecessary severity.

Wherever restraint may become necessary, owing to the imperfect adaptation of the building, or to a want of sufficient attendants, the most simple means should be selected. On such an occasion, I do not know of any constraint which would be preferable to that of seclusion in a darkened room. In this Asylum when a patient misconducts himself, he is immediately removed to the Refractory Patients' Gallery, where he remains until he has pledged himself that his future conduct shall be more orderly. This is the only method I employ to induce habits of self-control. A MANIAC IS SELDOM KNOWN TO BREAK HIS WORD.

Violent cases would be extremely rare in all Asylums, if the no-restraint system were generally adopted: as would suicides also, if, in conjunction with the above, Dormitories and Night-watches were established; but to dispense with restraint altogether such must be the case, or the attempt would be attended with extreme danger. Without the Dormitories and Night-watches it would be necessary to restrain such as exhibited a tendency to suicide. Under this system, i. e. the no-restraint system, cases of insensibility to natural calls would be seldom met with: to ensure the non-existence of such cases, the individuals must be removed from their own homes on the first appearance of the malady, or as soon afterwards as is practicable; before such habits have been induced by the use of the strait-waistcoat or other instruments which confine the fingers, and thus disable the patient from assisting himself on natural occasions.

I forgot to mention, when speaking of the Watch-room, that we have a clock fixed in this room which shows each time that the Watchman has been off duty. Should he sleep even a quarter of an hour during the night, it is pointed out˙ on the clock:—the Watchman is therefore compelled to be watchful. By this means the system of watching has been properly carried into effect. This clock is one of the most ingenious con-trivances you can imagine, and ensures watchfulness completely.

With your kind indulgence, I will trespass on your time and patience only a little longer, while I take a brief view of the *obstacles* to the practical execution of this, my theory. These obstacles do not arise from the nature of the cases—no, not in any one instance; neither are they in any instance *insurmountable*. What then are they? *First*,—The expense of providing a building having suitable apartments, Galleries, Dormitories, separate Sleeping Rooms, with Airing Courts, Pleasure Grounds, Gardens, and Walks:—and such ample remuneration of Attendants, as may ensure persons of character and respectability. But here it may be truly said, ' If a thing is worth doing at all, it is worth doing well!' If it be worth while to provide an Asylum

M 2

for the Insane, it is worth while also to render that Asylum complete for its purposes; otherwise the main objects of the Charity, viz.—the restoration of the afflicted inmates to sanity or providing for their comfort if irrecoverable—fall at once to the ground, and the Asylum becomes a mere prison.

Secondly,—The prejudice which this plan (as has been the case with every improvement on its first introduction) has to encounter. What! Let loose a Madman! Why he will tear us to pieces! Look a moment at the facts. The following Table, conjoined with the fact, that no serious accident has occurred under this system, will, I think, remove this idea from the mind of any impartial person.

NUMBER OF SUICIDES AND THEIR APPARENT CONNEXION WITH RESTRAINTS.

Date of House-Surgeon's Appointment.	Period Included.	Number of Patients Treated.	Number of Suicides.	Proportion of Suicides.	Rate of Coercion.
April 26, 1820.	10½ years	334	2	1 in 167	Maximum
Oct. 14, 1830.	3½ yrs. ⎱ 4¾ yrs.	173 ⎱ 242*	2 ⎱ 5	1 in 86½ ⎱ 1 in 48½	Medium
April 9, 1834.	1¼ yr. ⎰	120 ⎰	3 ⎰	1 in 40 ⎰	
July 8, 1835.	3½ years	246	0	0 in 246	Minimum

* From this total 51 have been deducted, being the number left in the house at the time of the third house-surgeon's appointment, and therefore necessarily counted as under treatment both of himself and his predecessor.

On comparing this Table with the Tables of Restraints, and from a knowledge of the circumstance that an effective system of watchfulness has only been introduced into the Asylum within the two or three last years,—it will appear that, without such a system of watchfulness,

A maximum of restraints is more safe than a medium.

With such a system of watchfulness, a minimum of restraints is more safe than either.

It must be borne in mind, that the attendants are or should be tall, and powerful in appearance. A diminutive person would be liable to be attacked: not so with the former; for a lunatic is perfectly aware (as is a sane person) with whom he has to deal. The attendants should be able to keep control without even the appearance of anger, and their demeanour and directions should be firm and decisive: nevertheless, this firmness must be always tempered with kindness; for a maniac may be drawn, when ill usage would but irritate him. I have never at any time had the slightest difficulty in calming a patient when he has been apparently in a state bordering on violence. I have been threatened several times, but never met with any injury. I have always been able to withdraw their attention, and they have generally afterwards expressed their regret for any roughness of their conduct towards me. One or two kind expressions I have generally found sufficient to assuage any feelings of anger or of violence ; and much will always depend on the demeanour of the Superintendent, as well as of the attendants.

Thirdly,—The unwillingness of attendants, nurses, &c., to undertake the increased trouble, which this system requires. Here I have found my greatest difficulty; and I know of no way of surmounting it, except by an ample remuneration of such persons. It is stated truly in the Report of this year, that " it is in the power of an unwilling officer to make any improvements fail in practice." When a patient is under restraint, it saves them the trouble of watching him: they can enjoy themselves at leisure, and play at cards, or otherwise amuse themselves as they please. Such was the case formerly, but cannot be tolerated under the new system. Their whole time and attention are now required for the patients.

I protest therefore, beforehand, against any failure in practice arising from unwillingness, inexperience, want of address, or impatience, on the part of any Officer, being converted into an argument against the system. Failures, if any should occur, will arise from one or other of the above causes, and not from the impracticability of the system itself. If others should not succeed in pursuing this plan, I shall have no fear of failure myself; as I feel confident that with a properly constructed building, and a sufficient number of tall, strong, well-remunerated, and *willing* attendants, I could introduce and act upon the system in any Asylum in the kingdom.

Shall then a plan, which has for its object the amelioration of the condition of an afflicted class of our fellow-creatures, and a more humane treatment of them, together with a better prospect of restoring them to the possession of that noblest gift of God, without which man sinks into a more abject state of misery and degradation than the beasts which perish—shall such a plan want advocates? I know it will not. I feel confident that it only requires to be made known, to be duly appreciated. Show its success, and humanity will compel its adoption. The Legislature of our Country deem not the welfare, the comfort, and happiness of any portion of the people, a subject unworthy of its consideration: and if instruments of cruelty are in the habitations which assume the names of a Refuge, an Asylum, a Retreat from misery and woe, let the Government, (when convinced of its practicability) banish them by law for ever! Let not the deeds done in an Asylum, render its very name a mockery. Let it be indeed a Refuge from distress; an Asylum, not in name, but in deed and in truth:—a place where the sufferer may be shielded from injury and insult—where his feelings may not be uselessly wounded, nor his innocent wishes wantonly thwarted. Here let him seek, and seek not in vain, that peace and comfort which are denied him in the paths he has formerly trod. Here let him repose until the light begin to dawn on his benighted mind, and he confess with heartfelt joy and gratitude, that the day he entered a Lunatic Asylum was indeed a blessed day!

On the conclusion of the Lecture, the President of the Mechanics' Institution, Sir E. Ff. Bromhead, Bart., F.R.S., L. and E., who is also a Vice-President of the Lincoln Asylum, offered some illustrative remarks on the subject of the Lecture, confirmatory of his own observation at the Asylum, of the soundness of the no-restraint theory. He then submitted to the meeting a formal vote of thanks to the Lecturer, which was carried in a manner most truly gratifying to his feelings.

APPENDIX.

(Appendix A.)

Opinions of Dr CHARLESWORTH upon the subject of restraint *prior* to the Author's connection with the Lincoln Lunatic Asylum, in July, 1835.

1828.—*Remarks on the Treatment of the Insane, &c.*

By E. P. CHARLESWORTH, M.D.—London: C. and J. Rivington.—" The modes of coercion are those which will excite least uneasiness, and have been most frequently a leathern belt, or a chain round the waist, with iron manacles for the wrists, attached to the belt or chain by a small chain a few inches long.

" For patients who tear their clothes, the ' muff' is generally employed. Perhaps leather used in the dress of these patients might occasionally supersede the necessity of restraint.

" Some cases require the use of the strait-waistcoat ; or, to prevent violent kicking, a restraint for the legs, called ' hobbles,' which allow the action of walking ; but these and the strait-waistcoat are comparatively little employed. The average number of patients under personal restraint, may be stated at from one to three in forty; sometimes not one for several weeks together.

" The restraints employed have been almost entirely at the discretion of the Director (House-Surgeon, or Medical Super-

intendent), always under his superintendence, and under the
eye of the physician and weekly visitor, whose attendance is
frequent and casual."—Pp. 16 and 17.

From the Minutes of the Asylum:

1832. *July* 16.—" Ordered, that buckskin and round-
cornered buckles be used for the hobbles.

" That a leathern belt, for temporary security of patients
becoming suddenly violent, be kept in the attendants' rooms."

July 23.—Resolved," That a pair of quarter boots (suggested
by Dr Charlesworth), with rings fixed to the soles, be procured as a night restraint for patients requiring the same."

1832.—*July* 31.—Physician's Report.—" It should be a
fixed principle in the construction of all instruments of
restraint, to prevent, as much as possible, the capability of the
patients to effect any injurious change of their position, or
otherwise to increase their severity. An insane patient will
act, while under a paroxysm, not only as if he were insensible of pain, but even as if he preferred a state of suffering
which would be found intolerable under ordinary circumstances. Multiplied instances, some of them very extraordinary, could be adduced in proof; and the pathological
inductions to which this fact would appear to lead, may
perhaps hereafter throw additional light upon the medical
history of insanity.

" *With regard to the ' fixing on' of the instruments of
restraint, nothing can prevent the dangers of negligence on the
part of the attendants in securing the locks,* or what is much
more common, the distressing severity of over caution in
tightening the straps, &c., *except minute and continually
repeated personal examination by the superior officers in each
individual instance, and especially of the cases left for the
night.*"

" (*Signed,*) E. P. CHARLESWORTH."

1834, *August* 11.—House-Visitor's Report.—" Examining the condition of the instruments (restraint) and fitting of the attendants' keys, I have found them all quite clean, but several out of order, as regards the locks and screws and keys. My notice of them would have led to their immediate regulation and repair, which is required to be attended to every Saturday; but *I would beg first to suggest that such of the wristlocks as are fastened by the tedious process of screwing, should be laid aside and replaced by others acting with spring-locks,* constructed, if practicable, with the inner surface made circular instead of oblong. This form would prevent the patients from inflicting intentional injury on themselves, as they not unfrequently have been known to do, by forcing the long diameter of the wrist across the shorter diameter of the manacle."

" (*Signed,*) GEO. MARR, Visitor."

1834, *August* 18. — " The Visitor's Report having been read : — Ordered, That the furnishing committee do take measures for procuring improved wristlocks for day and night use."

1834, *December* 29.—" Ordered, That one pair of night shoes (Dr Charlesworth's quarter boots for confining the feet) for male patients, and two pairs for females, be procured."

1835, *April.* — Eleventh Annual Report. — " A further review of the instruments of restraint has reduced them to four simple methods, viz. :

Day, 1.—The wrists secured by a flexible connection with a belt round the waist.

2.—The ancles secured by a flexible connection with each other, so as to allow of walking exercise.

Night, 3.—One or both wrists attached by a flexible connection to the sides of the bed.

4.—The feet placed in night-shoes, similarly attached to the foot of the bed.

The object of restraint is not punishment but security.

(*Signed,*) T. MANNERS SUTTON, Chairman.

(Appendix B.)

Proceedings of the Lincoln Lunatic Asylum with reference to non-restraint, and opinions of Dr CHARLESWORTH on the subject *subsequently* to the Author's connection with that Institution. Publication and Reviews of the Author's Lecture, &c.

1836, *March* 21.—12th Annual Report.—" Three successive months (excepting one day) have now elapsed without the occurrence of a single instance of restraint in this establishment : and out of thirty-six weeks that the House-Surgeon (Mr. R. G. Hill) has held his present situation, twenty-five whole weeks (excepting two days) have been passed without any recourse to such means, and even without one instance of confinement to a separate room."

(Signed,)   " R. PRETYMAN, Chairman."

1837, *April* 12.—13th Annual Report, by E. P. Charlesworth, M. D.—" The present House-Surgeon has expressed his own belief,* founded on experience in this house, that it may be possible to conduct an institution for the insane

---

* " It is worthy of remark, as Dr H. van Leeuwen was the first to point out, how carefully the Report guards against any misunderstanding of this matter. It does not merely say that the House-Surgeon has expressed his belief, &c., but that he has expressed '*his own*' belief—emphatically and exclusively ' *his own,*'—the belief of no one else at that time ; – and if the belief had been ' premature,' or ill-founded,—if the plan had proved abortive—the failure would have been emphatically and exclusively ' his own.' "—*Letter from the Rev. J. Daniel.*

without having recourse to the employment of any instruments of restraint whatsoever. He has certainly made a striking advance towards verifying this opinion by conducting the male (the completed) side of the house, without a solitary instance of such restraint, either by day or by night, during the course of the sixteen last months, and that applied only for about six hours, during his absence; nor is it impossible, when the buildings can be finished, that an example may be offered of an Asylum, in which undivided personal attention towards the patients shall be altogether substituted for the use of instruments.

"(*Signed,*)   W. M. PIERCE, Chairman."

1838, *March.*—Fourteenth Annual Report, by E. P. Charlesworth, M.D.—" There is now an increased confidence that the anticipations of the last year may be fulfilled, and that ' an ' example may be offered of a public Asylum, in which undi- ' vided personal attention towards the patients shall be ' altogether substituted for the use of instruments of restraint.' The bold conception of pushing the mitigation of restraint to the extent of actually and formally abolishing the practice, mentioned in the last Report as due to Mr Hill, the House-Surgeon, seems to be justified by the following abstract of a statistical Table,* showing the rapid advance of the abatement of restraints in this Asylum, under an improved construction of the building, night-watching, and attentive supervision. We may venture to affirm, that this is the first frank statement of the common practice of restraints, hitherto laid before a British public.

" Number of the patients restrained, and of the instances and hours of restraint, in eight successive years and nine months,

---

* " This Table was prepared by Mr Hill, who since his appointment in July, 1835, has, on this, as well as every other occasion, faithfully and unsparingly exerted himself to serve the interests of the institution. It is in the power of an unwilling officer to make any improvements fail in practice."

as extracted from the Register of Restraints, established March 16th, 1829, on the plan required by Law in Scotland.

Year.	Total number of Patients in the house.	Total number of Patients Restrained.	Total number of instances of Restraint.	Total number of Hours passed under Restraint.
1829 from March 16th	72	39	1727	20,423
1830	92	54	2364	27,113¾
1831	70	40	1004	10,880
1832	81	55	1401	15,671½
1833	87	44	1109	11,003½
1834	100	45	647	6,597
1835	108	28	323	2,874
1836	115	12	39	384
1837	130	2	3	28
1838	158	0	0	0

" This striking progress of amelioration affords good encouragement for persevering in a system so successfully commenced; and the more so, as a corresponding decrease of violence, accidents, and revolting habits, has accompanied the change.

" (Signed,)   E. P. CHARLESWORTH, Chairman."

1838, *June* 21.—Delivered Lecture on the Total Abolition of Restraint, at the Lincoln and Lincolnshire Mechanics' Institution.—Present, Sir E. Ff. Bromhead, Bart., in the Chair.

1838, Nov. 26. — Dr Charlesworth's Letter-testimonial to myself.—" He (Mr Hill) has diligently applied all the means of amelioration placed at his disposal, and in so doing has *conceived and effected results honourable to himself, and beyond the hopes of the board. The practice of restraint and coercion has disappeared under his management.*

" (Signed,)   E. P. CHARLESWORTH, M.D.,
Senior Physician of the Asylum."

1838, *November* 27.—Dr Cookson's Letter-testimonial to myself.—" He has, during his stay with us, *so completely substituted* a system of strict supervision, for the old system of restraint, that the latter has in our establishment become *entirely obsolete.*

" (*Signed,*)   W. D. COOKSON, M.D.,
Physician to the Lincoln Lunatic Asylum."

1839, *April* 13.—Published Lecture.

1839, *May* 15.—Review of Lecture in ' Lincoln Standard,' by Sir E. Ff. Bromhead, Bart.; revised by Dr. Charlesworth. —" It is not often that a provincial town has produced a work of this description, a work which may fairly lay claim to an European character, as forming a most marked era in the interesting subject on which it treats.   Mr Hill had, for some time, successfully carried into operation at our Asylum the total abolition of all restraint, and all severity, before he presented himself to the public as the deliverer of a lecture on the subject.   The Mechanics' Institution of this City has been of eminent service in giving a literary tone even to classes, whom want of opulence has excluded from the full benefits of regular education; but the opening which it has afforded for the occasional delivery of interesting lectures by its members, is not the least important.   In this lecture, Mr Hill exhibits a frightful picture of the ancient abuses universally inflicted on the insane, until the benevolent Pinel made an inroad on this domain of cruelty.   He began what Mr Hill has completed; the graphic description of some of Pinel's cases might touch the coldest heart; and some of the cases brought forward by Mr Hill, from the store of his own experience, are also of a very touching and affecting character.   The receptacles for the insane were formerly deemed places of safe keeping for wild beasts, in which cure was never dreamt of, except as the result of accident, and in which the most horrid and painful modes of confinement, amidst loathsome dirt, cold, and hunger, and frequent blows, was systematically practised, that the keepers (as the attendants were termed) might riot in debauchery, free from all concern and trouble about their

N

victims. The public will bear this no longer; the atrocities at Bethlem, York, and Warburton's, have awakened indignant sympathy, so that kindness is now universally professed, while the public eye is excluded with a kind of jealous dismay, lest forsooth the lunatic should be distressed by it. At Lincoln, the Boards resolutely set about to ameliorate the treatment, and have confirmed the remark, ' were every one to see the whole effects, mediate and immediate, present and remote, even of trifling acts of good' or evil, his mind would, on many occasions, be filled with delight or remorse.' The Governors *never expressed a wish for the extinction of restraints—they never expected it, not one of them deemed it possible;* they did all the good they could in a proper direction, they mitigated evil. They elected an honest, firm, sensible, and benignant medical man as a resident officer, they placed every possible facility in his way, and this honest and good man found himself landed triumphantly on an unhoped for territory. He had much to struggle with—the character of visionary humanity—the underplot of reluctant servants, who found every step in his progress a trespass on their own repose; and it may be considered most fortunate for mankind that no unlucky *apropos* accident blasted the plan for ever."

1839, *October* 9.—Entry in Governor's Memorandum Book. —" The entire absence of restraint still continues, *to the high honour of the House-Surgeon.*

" (Signed,)   EDW. FF. BROMHEAD,
W. M. PIERCE,
E. P. CHARLESWORTH."

1840, *November* 6.—Sir E. Ff. Bromhead's Letter-testimonial, addressed to the Chairman of the Lunatic Asylum, Bodmin.—" Thurlby Hall, Newark, Nov. 6, 1840. Sir, I have great pleasure in certifying my opinion of the probity, zeal, good temper, and solid judgment of Mr R. G. Hill, shown for several years as House-Surgeon of the Lincoln

Asylum. Having myself, for a very long period, paid much attention to this Asylum, the County Prison, and other public institutions, I can declare that I have not yet met with any officer so little disposed to content himself with formal duty, nor any who seemed more to take a deep personal interest in his duty. It is most honourable to him, that when I was in the chair on Mr Hill's retiring from office, the vote of regret for his loss, and thanks for his services, passed the Board unanimously, though the opponents of *his* system of throwing aside the strait-waistcoat and chains were then present. Most unhappily, this great improvement has been deemed a rebuke to the practice of Mr Hill's predecessors, and the practice of other houses, and has drawn much acrimonious exaggeration and even misstatement against the practice, and, finally, as might be expected, some hostility to the *author* from the party favourable to instrumental restraint and their friends.

" I have the honour to be, Sir, your very obedient servant,
" EDW. FF. BROMHEAD."

1841, *January* 3.—Physician's Report.—" The bold position taken by Mr Hill in his publication on the non-restraint system, assuming the practicability of a total abolition of instrumental restraint, was not less sensible than sound. The present House-Surgeon has taken a similar position as regards the abolition of solitary confinement, and I trust he will succeed in his object, *as Mr Hill has done in his own.*

" (*Signed,*) E. P. CHARLESWORTH."

1849, *July* 30. — Twenty-fifth Annual Report. —" The cases diminished with unexpected rapidity, and sometimes weeks or months elapsed without any case at all; at last, under these circumstances, the idea occurred to Mr Hill, that *no case of the kind whatsoever need exist :* and, in the practice, he was determinedly supported by the Boards, through every species of opposition, exaggeration, and misrepresentation, within the institution and without.

" (*Signed,*) E. FF. BROMHEAD, Vice-President."

1850, *August* 16.—Extract from Dr. Charlesworth's speech at the dinner of the Provincial Medical and Surgical Association, at Hull, as reported in the 'Eastern Counties' Herald.'

" The *real honour* of first introducing the system, is due to Mr Hill."*

---

* As Dr Charlesworth subsequently stated that he " doubted " whether he expressed himself in these exact terms, or not, I have thought it advisable to corroborate the fact by reference to other evidence. The 'Lancet,' whose own reporter was present, thus reports it :—" The real honour belonged to Mr Hill, of the Lincoln Asylum."—The 'Provincial Medical Journal,' the organ of the society, made a similar statement, from their own reporter. In the ' Lincolnshire Times,' the following account is given of the proceedings of that day :—" At a meeting of the Provincial Medical and Surgical Association, held at the Public Rooms at Hull, on Thursday last, Dr Horner in the chair, supported on his right by Sir C. Hastings, M.D., Drs W. and J. Conolly, E. P. Charlesworth, Esq., M.D., R. G. Hill, Esq., and about a hundred more medical gentlemen, Sir Charles Hastings took the opportunity of proposing the health of Dr John Conolly, and alluded to the testimonial about to be presented to him for his great services in carrying out the principles of *non-coercion* at the Lunatic Asylum at Hanwell.—Dr Conolly, in reply, stated that it was a great pride to him that he had found out that system which mitigated much of the suffering attendant upon *insanity;* but that he only followed, and was not the author of that most valuable and humane system ; that the merit was due to Dr Charlesworth and Mr Hill, who originated it at the Asylum at Lincoln. He therefore felt great pleasure in making this acknowledgement before his medical brethren, and he begged to propose the health of Dr Charlesworth, and Mr Hill, who was the Surgeon to the Lincoln Asylum. Dr Charlesworth, in returning thanks, said he was glad of the opportunity, like his friend Dr Conolly, of acknowledging that he, as well as the Doctor, was not the originator of the system referred to ; but he felt equal pleasure in acknowledging publicly, that the introduction of the system, and the merit of it, was due to Mr Hill.—Mr Hill also returned thanks, and stated that he felt exceedingly proud in having awarded to him, before his medical brethren, the credit to which he believed he was entitled."—' Lincolnshire Times,' August 13th, 1850.

Extract from Dr H. Munro's Letter to the Author.—" Hull, March 18th, 1851.—Being one of the Stewards of that dinner, and having on my left hand Dr Charlesworth, and yourself next to him, I can distinctly recollect the remarks made by both of you. After the admirable speech of Dr Conolly, in which he referred to the labours of Dr Charlesworth and yourself, with all that kindly feeling so much the characteristic of that gentleman, Dr Charlesworth at once replied, in language as honourable as it was praiseworthy, that the real honour of discovering the improved treatment of the insane belonged to his colleague, Mr Hill."

Extract from Dr James Heygate's Letter, addressed to R. S. Harvey, Esq.—
" Derby, March 18th, 1851.—I cannot, however, resist the pleasure of bearing
my testimony to the fact of that gentleman (Mr Hill) being the originator of the
non-restraint system. I have a vivid recollection of all the circumstances connected therewith."

Dr Robertson's evidence, in reply to the enquiries of the Testimonial Committee,
will be found in Appendix (D.)

(Appendix C.)

EXTRAORDINARY attack upon the Author's claims as the originator of the non-restraint system by Sir Edward Ffrench Bromhead, Bart., a Vice-President of the Lincoln Lunatic Asylum, in direct opposition to all his own previous testimony; and replies thereto.

From the 'LANCET,' *November* 23, 1850.

ON THE DISUSE OF INSTRUMENTS OF RESTRAINT IN LUNACY,

WITH AN ACCOUNT OF THE PROCEEDINGS FOR THIS PURPOSE IN THE LINCOLN LUNATIC ASYLUM.

[Letter from Sir E. F. Bromhead, Bart.]

TO THE EDITOR OF THE 'LANCET.'

Sir,—It is a matter of gratification to find that the disuse of instrumental restraint in the treatment of the insane is now so far confirmed, as a principle, that the history of its rise, progress, and establishment, has become a matter of interest. No individual can exclusively claim the merit. To Pinel and others on the continent, every honour is due ; but they never made any approach to the total disuse of instruments.

At the Lincoln Asylum, the earlier system was restraint, under the most oppressive and revolting forms. It was not in any way disguised, but was rather considered in practice a proof of care, vigorous management, and rigorous precaution.

In October, 1821, the Boards, under the advice of Dr Charlesworth, the present senior physician, began to attack this system, on the principle of attempting to supersede instrumental restraint, and also of wholly disusing the more mischievous instruments, as the strait-waistcoat ; and of reducing the forms of such as remained to a state that might, as far as possible, restrain the patient without producing irritation, or preventing the proper use of his limbs.

The number of the instruments was reduced to a low scale; a separate depôt, under the key of the house-surgeon, was provided for them, that they should not be too conveniently at hand ; a " register" was required to be kept, in which daily entry was made of the commencement and end of each instance of the use of any instrument; and various contrivances were adopted to obviate their necessity. A sufficient staff of attendants was placed at the disposal of the house-surgeon; those attendants were exonerated from all other duties, and were selected of such a stature as would secure them from the contempt and attack of patients disposed to violence.

The additional trouble attending the imposition of instruments led them to look less and less to that resource; and, when a patient was strangled in the night by a strait-waistcoat, its future use (though declared indispensable) was instantly found unnecessary, on an order that an attendant should sit up all night with each patient said to require it. The irritating effects of fermented drink were removed, under the substitution of an invigorating animal diet. Various amusements and occupations were introduced ; the building was enlarged, and watch-dormitories were formed, and the airing grounds were extended and improved. It was also distinctly made known to each house-surgeon, on his accession, that his ability and competency would be considered as tested by the extent to which he could carry out the disuse of instruments.

It would be tedious to enumerate all the resources from time to time placed at the disposal of the successive house-surgeons. These, under the influence and atmosphere of a general amelioration in all the other departments, produced a diminution on the " register of restraint" at a steady accelerated rate.

At this point, Mr Hill became house-surgeon, in July, 1835, and, with great good temper, good feeling, and good sense, most honestly, efficiently, and perseveringly carried out and applied all the means placed at his disposal by the Board. He had found the instances of restraint reduced by his predecessors in the proportion of from seven to one, and he rapidly reduced that proportion to a still lower limit.

Presently he passed a period of several successive months without the single application of an instrument; and eventually had the courage to broach the original and invaluable idea, " that the use of instruments might be WHOLLY dispensed with."

The Board received this suggestion with much satisfaction, but still considered it a matter of experiment to be worked out by induction on every variety of case, and over a large period of time ; and they expressed a determination to give him every support in this great experiment, in the face of every misrepresentation and hostile annoyance which the idea drew upon the Board and upon himself.

At length the Board came to this conclusion—that no cautious and prudent person could possibly declare, *a priori*, that there was no extreme case, among the infinite phases of lunacy, in which an instrument might not be applied without injury to the individual, and, perhaps, even with some advantage : but the Board, on further induction. took the new ground, that if any such case did exist, it had been wholly out of their experience, and must be of the rarest occurrence, and probably produced by the very system itself; and that the benefit, if any, could not compensate for the admission of a principle so deadly in its operation, and so obviously open to indefinite extension and abuse. Even the old system of flagellation itself might be well defended, on the possible existence of benefit in some exceptional cases. So cautious, indeed, were the Boards, that the practice was left open to the discretion and responsibility of the house surgeons, and was not formally abolished *by rule* till July, 1843.

Such is the history of this matter at the Lincoln Asylum, and I claim for myself, and other governors, the merit of having supported Dr Charlesworth, the present senior-physician, through every obstruction and misrepresentation, and the treachery of some unwilling agents, in his indefatigable efforts to obviate the necessity of instruments, by the substitution of a long series of resources and precautions. I also claim for myself the merit of having laid before the public, in many of the Reports, the history of its proceedings, argued and defended, partly from the valuable conversation and suggestions of that intelligent and benevolent individual, and partly also from my own researches.

The crowning merit, however, of the diffusion and establishment of the new system over the face of England, and of the civilised world, is eminently due to Dr Conolly, and to a few other heads of extensive institutions. The principle might have been born at Lincoln, and expired in the place of its birth, on a too limited induction of cases, if that great and good man—an honour to this nation—had not brought his genius to bear upon the question, on the broader and more public field of Hanwell. There he had gigantic difficulties to contend with ; a formidable and paralyzing opposition ; the disinclination of the Commissioners ; and he had to call into action every resource of genius, energy, and invention, to meet an infinite variety of difficult cases, and details. Neither ought we to forget the enlightened and public-spirited support of an influential medical press, as an auxiliary in this humane movement.

E. F. BROMHEAD,

Vice-President of the Lincoln Asylum.

From the 'LANCET,' *Dec.* 21, 1850.

THE DISUSE OF INSTRUMENTS OF RESTRAINT IN LUNACY.

[Letter from Mr R. Gardiner Hill.]

"SUUM CUIQUE."

TO THE EDITOR OF THE 'LANCET.'

Sir,—Will you permit me, through your valuable journal, to make a few observations on the statements put forth by Sir Edward Ffrench Bromhead in his letter on the disuse of instruments of restraint in lunacy. At the commencement of his letter he says "no individual can exclusively claim the merit" of this disuse. Now, Sir, without attempting to disparage the just claims of any one to the merit of attacking the old system of cruelty, or of acting upon a system of mitigation of restraint, or subsequently, to the merit of carrying out a previously announced system of non-restraint, I will only ask you to compare these words with another paragraph of Sir Edward's letter, wherein he distinctly and emphatically says, that it was Mr Hill who "had the courage to broach the original and invaluable idea that ' the use of instruments might be wholly dispensed with!'" Who, then, Sir, I ask, can claim the merit of this "original idea" but myself? That Lincoln was the birth-place of the abolition of restraint is now universally allowed. The simple question is, then, with whom did it originate? Let facts and documents, not assertions, answer. It must have originated either with the governors, the visiting physicians, or the house-surgeon, of the Asylum. It did not originate with the governors of the Asylum, for they have distinctly stated that "the *bold conception* of pushing the mitigation of restraint to the extent of actually and formally abolishing the practice" is due to Mr Hill, the house-surgeon," (see Report, 1838). It did not originate with the physicians, for the resident house-surgeon had the control and management of restraint, subject to the general directions of the institution, whose system was that of mitigation; and Dr

Charlesworth, at the dinner of the Provincial Medical and Surgical Society at Hull, distinctly disclaimed this merit for himself, and candidly and honourably, as well as truly, assigned it to me. With all this agrees what Sir Edward F. Bromhead says, that "the *original* and invaluable idea" was broached by Mr Hill. True; the idea *is* an invaluable one, as proved by its results; it was, as Sir Edward truly says, "*original*," and "it was broached by Mr Hill." This is clear and decisive. It originated with the house-surgeon, and that house-surgeon was myself.

Can it be the same Sir E. F. Bromhead, who, notwithstanding the highly complimentary manner in which he states the fact, says, almost in the same breath, "No individual can exclusively claim the merit"!

It is on this account, Sir, that I have presumed to request so much of your space. I should not, indeed, have troubled you with any further remarks of mine, did it not appear, from those words, that while the honour of broaching the original and invaluable idea of total abolition cannot be withheld from me, there is (strange to say) an evident wish to detract from the merit of it, by representing it as a result of the labours of others. I do not wish, as I have said, to under-value these labours; but notwithstanding them, all that was thought of was a milder system of restraint, the disuse of some of the severer instruments, and a greater consideration for the comfort and well-being of the patients. "Total abolition" was not even hoped for by the most sanguine and philanthropic, until I announced it as a principle, and justified its soundness by its results.

It appears from the "Register of Restraints" of the Lincoln Asylum, established in the early part of 1829, that from that date to Dec. 31, 1835, no less than 95,875 hours were passed under instrumental restraint by different individuals! To such a degree was instrumental restraint used, under a system of mitigation, and immediately previous to my appointment as house-surgeon! The following table will show the result of the treatment during that period, and the percentage of recoveries and deaths, as affected by restraint:—

Patients discharged from the Books.	Having been under Restraint.	Not having been under Restraint.	Number of Hours passed under Res raint.	Average Numuer of Hours under Restraint.	Per-centage as affected by		Per-centage of Suicides.	Per-centage of Deaths from Ma- niacal Exhaustion.
					Restrnt.	Non-Restrnt.		
Recovered or Improved .... } 161	65	96	23,616	363	40.37	59.62		
Dead 52	44	8	48,394	1.100	84.61	15.38	11.11	9.61
Removed during treatment, escaped, and remaining in the House .... } 110	78	32	23,865	306				
Totals 323	187	136	95,875		57.89	42.10		

After carefully weighing the results indicated by this table, no one can be surprised at my attempting to introduce a new system. Even the most improved instruments occasioned, under the writhings and struggles of the maniac, the most agonizing pain and suffering, and fearfully impeded recovery.

With respect to the support alleged to be given to Dr Charlesworth, through obloquy, misrepresentation, and abuse— alas! Sir, it was the unfortunate individual who now addresses you that bore the brunt of this hard usage. As the system was essentially mine, so was the opposition which it called forth. And truly, no species of persecution, short of absolute bodily torture was left untried by various opponents of the new system. Within the Asylum itself, and its weekly board-room, so strongly was this spirit manifested, that at last no resource was left me but to resign an appointment, the scanty emolument of which was my sole support, and to the efficiency of which I had devoted all the energies of my mind, and almost all my hard-earned savings. The Report of 1849 will show that the violence of the attack was upon me, not upon the visiting physicians nor the governors.

Subsequent to my resignation, I drew up a Report in defence of my system, and the Quarterly Board of Governors (July 1840) passed the following resolution:—" That the thanks of this General Board are due to Mr Hill, for his clear, convincing, and most satisfactory statement, and that the same, and the appendix, be entered upon the minutes of the Board, to accompany the evidence produced against the character of this establishment."

But perhaps the most important document I can refer to in support of my claim, and of Sir Edward Bromhead's knowledge of the individual to whom " exclusively " the merit of the total disuse of instruments is due, is the following letter of Sir E. F. Bromhead, addressed to the Chairman of the Lunatic Asylum, Bodmin, when the author was a Candidate for the office of Medical Superientendent of that Asylum.

"THURLBY HALL, Newark, Nov. 6, 1840.

" Sir,—I have great pleasure in certifying my opinion of the probity, zeal, good temper, and solid judgment of Mr R. G. Hill, shown for several years as House-Surgeon of the Lincoln Asylum. Having myself for a very long period paid much attention to this asylum, the County prison, and other public institutions, I can declare that I have not yet met with any officer so little disposed to content himself with formal duty, nor any who seemed more to take a deep personal interest in his duty. It is most honourable to him, that when I was in the chair on Mr Hill's retiring from office, the vote of regret for his loss, and thanks for his services, passed the Board unanimously, though the opponents of *his* system of throwing aside the strait-waistcoat and chains were then present. Most unhappily, this great improvement has been deemed a rebuke to the practice of Mr Hill's predecessors, and the practice of other houses, and has drawn much acrimonious exaggeration and even mis-statement against the practice ; and, finally, as might be expected, some hostility to the author * from the parties favourable to instrumental restraint and their friends.

I have the honour to be, Sir,

Your very obedient servant,

EDWARD FF. BROMHEAD."

Sir,—I almost fear to advert to the concluding paragraph of Sir Edward's letter, lest it should be thought by any one that I do so in an invidious spirit. I do not deny the merit due to that great and good man, Dr Conolly, of carrying out the non-restraint system, through gigantic difficulties, on the broader and more public field of Hanwell. But the merit of carry out a system is one thing; the merit of *originating* it, is another: let each one bear his own fair proportion in the scale. If it be an honour to a man to carry out a humane and benevolent system for the good of his fellow-creatures, it cannot be otherwise than an honour to have announced that system, to have predicted its blessings and its success.

Should, however, my exertions in the common cause of humanity meet with no other reward, they have had *one* encouraging stimulus—the honourable mention of them by that mighty engine, the press. Even the very hostile attacks made upon the system by various ephemeral publications, only contributed eventually to settle it upon a firmer basis, by calling forth advocates of the highest power and influence, whose approval was at once the earnest and the guarantee of success.—Apologizing for the length of this communication,

I am, Sir,

Your obedient and much-obliged Servant,

ROBERT GARDINER HILL.

Lincoln, Dec. 3, 1850.

---

* " No individual can exclusively claim the merit."—Letter from Sir E. F. Bromhead to the 'Lancet,' Nov. 28, 1850.

From the ' LANCET,' *Dec.* 21, 1850.

[*Letter from the Rev. Mr Daniel.*]

TO THE EDITOR OF THE 'LANCET.'

Sir,—I am one of those who have watched with pleasure the rapid progress and adoption of humane measures in the management of our Asylums. We have only to refer to the authentic documents and reports of a period not yet out of memory, to see what a load of misery and suffering has thus been removed by the benevolent efforts of various energetic and talented individuals. The ingenuity, also, of many plans and contrivances, which have been gradually introduced to supersede the more cruel methods of instrumental restraint, is really surprising. The eminent men to whose genius and humanity these improvements are owing, deserve well of their country: let their names be had in everlasting honour.

On this ground, Sir, I rejoice to see that the persevering labours of such philanthropists as Dr Conolly are appreciated as they ought to be. His success in the large institution of Hanwell has demonstrated, beyond a doubt, the practicability of that unexpected climax of humanity in the treatment of the insane; the system of total abolition, or non-restraint. For the announcement of this " original and invaluable idea," as it is well described by Sir E. F. Bromhead in his interesting letter inserted in your journal of November 23rd, the world is indebted to my worthy friend and relative, Mr Robert Gardiner Hill, at that time House-Surgeon of the Lincoln Asylum; and a more faithful, honest, and zealous officer that institution never possessed. Originality, Sir, is the distinctive mark of genius ; and I will venture to say, that as much true genius was displayed in the mode of originating this improvement, as in any great discovery of modern times. The principle of the Lincoln Asylum was mitigation of restraint, so far as was deemed consistent with safety; and it was by a series of inductions, worthy of any great mind, and by living amongst the patients himself, and performing the duties of attendant, as well as

House-Surgeon, that Mr Hill arrived at the conclusion, that under a system of constant surveillance, with a suitable number of able and willing attendants, and in a properly-constructed building, "restraint is never necessary, never justifiable, but always injurious, in all cases of lunacy whatever."

I have witnessed, Sir, his zeal, his perseverance, his untiring energy; I have known, from the first, the yearning of his kind heart to relieve this species of human misery; and (I say it without disparagement to the just claims of others) I am sure that if ever there was a man who has deserved and earned a public testimonial to his merit, that man is Robert Gardiner Hill.—I am, Sir, yours faithfully—JOHN DANIELL,
Incumbent of East Ardsley, Yorkshire, and a
Subscriber to your Journal.
East Ardsley Parsonage, Wakefield, Dec. 4, 1850.

From the 'LANCET,' *Dec.* 28, 1850.
THE DISUSE OF INSTRUMENTS OF RESTRAINT IN LUNACY.
[*Letter from Sir E. F. Bromhead.*]
TO THE EDITOR OF THE 'LANCET.'

Sir,—Mr Gardiner Hill cannot think that I am acting unfairly towards him in adopting his own preface to his published lecture, as almost *verbatim* my view of his position with regard to the Lincoln Asylum.—E. F. BROMHEAD,
Vice-President of the Lincoln Asylum.

Preface to a Lecture on the Management of Lunatic Asylums and the Treatment of the Insane, delivered at the Mechanics' Institution, Lincoln, on the 21st of June, 1836, by Robert Gardiner Hill, Member of the Royal College of Surgeons, London, House-Surgeon of the Lincoln Lunatic Asylum.

" The object of the following lecture is simply to advocate the total abolition of severity, of every species and degree, as applied to patients in our Asylums for the insane, and with this view to show—first, that such abolition is in theory highly desirable ; and, secondly, that it is practicable, in proof of which assertions the present state of the Lincoln Lunatic Asylum is adduced.   There such a system is in actual and successful operation—the theory verified by the practice. It may be proper to state here, that the principle of mitigation of restraint, to the utmost extent that was deemed consistent with safety, was ever the principle pressed upon the attention of the Boards of the Lincoln Asylum by its humane and able physician, Dr Charlesworth.   At his suggestion, many of the more cruel instruments of restraint were long since destroyed, very many valuable improvements and facilities gradually adopted, and machinery set in motion, which has led to the unhoped for result of actual abolition, under a firm determination to work out the system to its utmost applicable limits. To his steady support under many difficulties, I owe chiefly the success which has attended my plans and labours.   He originated the requisite alterations and adaptations in the building, and threw every other facility in the way of accomplishing the object * * * * * The author is proud to have learned in such a school, and gladly owns the obligation.

"Lincoln Lunatic Asylum, April, 1839."

From the 'LANCET,' *January* 4, 1849.

DISUSE OF INSTRUMENTAL RESTRAINT IN LUNATIC ASYLUMS.

TO THE EDITOR OF THE 'LANCET.'

Sir,—There is nothing in the preface to my Lecture quoted by Sir E. F. Bromhead, which at all invalidates my claim to be the author of the total abolition or non-restraint system.   It only states, that " the principle of mitigation of restraint to the utmost extent that was deemed consistent with safety, was

P

ever the principle pressed upon the attention of the Boards of the Lincoln Asylum, by its humane and able physician, Dr Charlesworth ;"—that by the experience acquired in " working out this system to its utmost applicable limits," I became convinced that restraint was altogether unnecessary ;—that I announced this as a principle, and acted upon it with success ; that the " plans and labours " connected with " total abolition," or " non-restraint," were mine, and that Dr Charlesworth steadily assisted me in carrying out these plans, for which he had and has my sincere thanks.

Once more, allow me to prove my claims by reference to documents.

1. *Report of Lincoln Asylum*, 1837, *signed by W. M. Pierce.*—" The present House-Surgeon [Mr Hill] has expressed his own belief, founded on experience in this house, that it may be possible to conduct an institution for the insane without having recourse to the employment of any instruments of restraint whatsoever."

2. *The Report of* 1838, *signed by Dr Charlesworth, says, that the* " bold conception of pushing the mitigation of restraint " (the previous system of the Lincoln Asylum), " to the extent of absolutely and formally abolishing the practice," [my system] " is due to Mr Hill, the House-Surgeon."

3. *Extract from Dr Charlesworth's letter-testimonial to myself, dated November 26, 1838.*—" He " [Mr Hill] " has diligently applied all the means of amelioration placed at his disposal, and in so doing has *conceived and effected results* honourable to himself, and *beyond the hopes of the Board.*

" *The practice of restraint and coercion has disappeared under his management.*"

4. *From Dr Cookson's letter-testimonial to myself, dated November 27th, 1838.*—" He has during his stay with us so *completely substituted* a system of strict supervision for the old system of restraint, that the latter has in our establishment become *entirely obsolete.*"

5. *Extract from the Governors' Memorandum Book, Lincoln Asylum, Oct.* 9, 1839.—" The entire absence of restraint still continues, *to the high honour of the House-Surgeon.*

" (*Signed,*)   EDW. FF. BROMHEAD.

W. M. PIERCE.

E. P. CHARLESWORTH."

6. *Report of Lincoln Asylum,* 1849, *signed E. F. Bromhead.*—" The cases " [of restraint] " diminished with unexpected rapidity, and sometimes weeks or months elapsed without any case at all; at last, under these circumstances, the idea occurred to Mr Hill, *that no case of the kind whatsoever need exist;* and in the practice he was determinedly supported by the Boards, through every species of opposition, exaggeration, and misrepresentation, within the institution and without."

7. *Extract from Sir E. F. Bromhead's letter-testimonial, November 6th,* 1840.—" It is most honourable to him that when I was in the chair, on Mr Hill's retiring from office, the vote of regret for his loss, and thanks for his services, passed the Board unanimously, though the opponents of *his system* of throwing aside the strait-waistcoat and chains were then present. Most unhappily, this great improvement has drawn some hostility upon *the author* from the parties favourable to instrumental restraint."

8. *Extract from Dr Charlesworth's speech at the dinner of the Provincial Medical and Surgical Association at Hull, as reported in the* 'Eastern Counties Herald,' *August* 15, 1850.— " The *real honour* of first introducing the system is due to Mr Hill."

I trust that the above testimonies are sufficiently decisive of my claims.

I remain, Sir,

Your obliged and obedient Servant,

ROBERT GARDINER HILL.

Lincoln, Dec. 30, 1850.

From the 'LANCET,' *February* 1, 1851.

[*Letter from the Coroner of Lincoln.*]

TO THE EDITOR OF THE 'LANCET.'

Sir,—Controversy carried on in a spirit of fairness generally results in the public deriving the advantage.

I have, Sir, read in your journal some letters which have revived, in a useful manner, *the question of the non-restraint of the insane.*

The perusal of Sir Edward Ffrench Bromhead's letter occasioned much surprise, so much so, that in discussing its *points*, the question arose,—What object? What motive? *Cui bono?* To the two first, I will neither assume nor state an answer, because I might give a false one, or be led to attribute an unjust one; to the third, *cui bono?* I will venture one, and for which I thank Sir Edward—viz., that he has again called public attention to so vital a subject.

The erection, on the summit of our Cliffe Hill, of a spacious County Asylum for the insane, in which, *it is said*, the *system of restraint* is to be carried out, gives an increased interest to the question, not as to the *originator*, but as to the *merits* of the system.

To Mr Hill we are much indebted for his remarkably temperate letter, in reply to Sir Edward's. We have, Sir, daily advertisers in the London press, whose advertisements are headed " The Graphiologist," which means, I believe, " your character seen in your hand-writing." I will not undertake to say what of character may be understood by the mere *mechanical* act of *writing ;* but I can understand how, from epistolary composition, the calibre and temperament of the mind and the quality of the disposition may be judged of ; and if I may be allowed an opinion, I would say that the letter of Mr Hill displays a mind conscious that his case has a giant's power, but has also a benevolence that controls its use.

Since my residence in Lincoln, I have never heard the

question mooted as to *who* was the *originator* of the mild treatment of those, the most heavily afflicted by the destruction of their reason—that mighty *fulcrum* by which man is raised above all creation ; but on its first promulgation, I frequently heard its practicability disputed, and its author, Mr Hill, declared to be qualified for an admission patient. The great merit of being the *originator* of the *non-restraint system* was not only accorded to Mr Hill by the senior physician to the Asylum, Dr Charlesworth, but, to his honour will it be ever recorded, that no jealousy as to authorship ever arose; but with a vigorous mind, and with that indomitable perseverance —his *aura popularis*—he combated the opposition of his medical brethren, and overthrew the prejudices created by that opposition, until the late eminent and excellent man, Dr Cookson, junior, accorded his *converted* conviction in its favour. But not only was the triumph of a good system over a bad one achieved, but the *fame* of the Lincoln Lunatic Asylum has acquired strength in its progress.

The question of restraint or non-restraint is well worthy the attention and deep consideration of the directors or the governors of the new County Asylum; and also, as a question of *expense*, worthy the attention of the *rate-payers*. Let, therefore, the matter be well thought of. Mr Hill, in his temperate letter, has given some useful and opportune statistics, to which I would call the attention of the Governors. He states that in a given period, that of patients *under restraint* sixty-five have " recovered or improved," and forty-four have died; whereas, under *non-restraint*, ninety-six have " recovered or improved," and *only eight have died !* And under the classification of suicides I believe it is *as one hundred to nothing !*

By some it is urged, that the Lincoln Asylum being carried on on a small scale, furnishes no *positive* evidence for a general adoption of the system. Fortunately for the question, the results at Hanwell Asylum—which is much more extensive than the one now erecting in our County, the system under the superintendence of (as Mr Hill justly describes him) that " great and good man," Dr Conolly, demonstratively proves its efficacy, and that it *ought to influence* the decision of the Governors of the Lincoln County Asylum.

While on the subject of *contrast*, I would wish to call public attention to another interesting and important feature in the humane system of non-restraint : evidence is not required to prove the existence of a general horror and alarm at the idea of visiting an Asylum for the insane. A wall of partition, as thick as those of Troy, is erected in the public mind generally between the sane and the insane. Not so, Sir, in the Lincoln Lunatic Asylum; for at stated periods you will see childhood, from three years to thirteen ; puberty, from thirteen to twenty-one; and maturity, to eighty, mingling and co-mingling with the insane, unattended by fear, stimulated by confidence, and uniting with them in playfulness, or joining with them in amusements in the open grounds ! Is this, Sir, not a happy change from confinement in the dark, dank cells, into which too many have been placed? Is it any longer a problematical question, as to the *chances* of recovery, by the enjoyment of liberty instead of the strait-waistcoat, the wrist and leg-locks, &c. &c., worn under the restraint system ?

As the question has been thus again brought before the public, I trust *demonstrative* measures will be taken, and that, as it is really *a national question*, legislative interference shall be demanded, to render the system of non-restraint compulsory both in public and private Asylums.

I am, Sir, your obedient Servant,

JAMES HITCHINS,

Coroner for the City and County of Lincoln.

High street, Lincoln, Dec. 31, 1850.

(Appendix D.)

[Similar attack by the Rev. W. M. PIERCE, a
Governor of the Lincoln Lunatic Asylum,
also in direct opposition to all his own previous testimony; and replies thereto. Insi-
dious and indirect support of the attack by
Dr Charlesworth, contrary to all his former
statements.]

From the 'LANCET,' *February* 1, 1851.

DISUSE OF INSTRUMENTS OF RESTRAINT IN LUNACY.
THE CLAIMS OF MR R. GARDINER HILL.

[*Letter from a Governor of the Lincoln Asylum.*]

TO THE EDITOR OF THE 'LANCET.'

Sir,—As Mr Hill has brought forward my name, with
that of others, in support of his recent claim to have been the
author and originator of the non-restraint system in lunacy,
I beg leave distinctly to express my dissent from this assumption, however coloured by passages carefully gleaned without
reference to context, or the circumstances under which they
occurred. The true author and originator of the non-restraint
system is Dr Charlesworth. This gentleman was not satisfied
with the humane mitigation of Pinel, in France, and of the
Retreat in this kingdom. He avowedly insisted on the abolition
of restraint at the Lincoln Asylum, at whatever amount of inconvenience to the establishment, to the utmost possible extent
found consistent with personal safety. He set on foot a sys-
tematic course of progressive experiment, regularly reported to

the public, for the avowed purpose of ascertaining the utmost extent to which it was possible to dispense with instruments. He devised and organised, I think I may say, the whole of the arrangements necessary for carrying the experiment to a successful issue, and those were the very means by which the inevitable result was attained. The responsibility on the point of personal safety could not but rest with the resident officer, though that officer well knew that his humanity, ability, attention to duty, and even his personal courage, were estimated by the extent to which he reduced the number of exceptional cases; and he knew also that every exceptional case was viewed with the greatest distaste and suspicion by the superintending physician and the Boards. The exceptional cases diminished with an accelerated rapidity, as experience proved the safety and gave additional confidence to the establishment; and under Mr Hill's predecessor there was only, on an average, a single exceptional case per day, and sometimes not even a single case for weeks together. That gentleman left the institution for a better situation, and it cannot be doubted that had he continued a little longer in office that this single exceptional case, viewed with such jealousy by the Boards, must have disappeared, and Dr Charlesworth's experiments reached its inevitable result before Mr Hill's appointment. Mr Hill's merit has always been allowed with lavish generosity, even to overflowing, from his willingness to co-operate steadily with Dr Charlesworth, and to bear his share of the hostility which professional jealousy and personal enmity are everywhere ready to exhibit; and Mr Hill once declared himself 'proud to have learned in such a school.' Mr Hill can scarcely pretend that he had anything in the world to do with what preceded his appointment: it will scarcely be denied that Dr Charlesworth must have arrived at the result of his experiment without Mr Hill, though Mr Hill's name never could have been connected with the matter without Dr Charlesworth. Mr Hill had a single exceptional case to cope with, under every possible advantage, and, from the course of the experiment, the exceptional case was sometimes not seen for months, and then, at last, Mr Hill declared himself competent to cope with any case whatever. No one wishes to deprive him of this merit, though he unhappily did give way in a case shortly before his retiring, leaving his successor, in fact, the first who actually carried out the non-restraint system under the supervision of the physician and the Boards. In short, Mr Hill was an agent in an experiment to which he has not any claim whatever. He has, indeed, the justly-earned merit of being the first to conjecture a result, which his own subsequent failure proved to be premature, and which Dr Charlesworth was too cautious and philosophic to assume on inadequate induction.

As Mr Hill deals in extracts, I will request you to subjoin the following, from a report which he prides himself upon having been entered on the board-minutes of the Lincoln Asylum, July 8, 1840.

" On succeeding to the office of House-Surgeon to this institution, I found that the use of instruments of restraint had been dispensed with, frequently for days together, sometimes much longer, as shown in my publication. I watched the patients and the attendants closely, and at last came to the conclusion that if instruments could be dispensed with for weeks and months together, they might be dispensed with altogether. The House-Surgeon before my predecessor had thought necessary to restrain from six to seven patients daily. My predecessor reduced this number still lower, and had seldom more than one patient under restraint at one time. If the patients have, since my appointment, undergone numerous and daily abuses (as endeavoured to be impressed) for want of instrumental restraint, they must have been in the same manner abused during my predecessor's superintendence, for he reduced the number of restraints from seven to one, I merely from one to none."

I am, Sir, your obedient servant,

W. M. PIERCE, A.M.,

A Governor of the Lincoln Asylum for

more than twenty years.

West Ashby, Jan. 11, 1851.

From the 'LANCET,' *February* 1, 1851.

[*Letter from Dr Charlesworth.*]

TO THE EDITOR OF THE 'LANCET.'

Sir,—Mr Hill having quoted some expressions as used by me at a public meeting, I feel called upon to say that I doubt my having expressed myself in those exact terms, and that I certainly never contemplated the conclusion which he has drawn, however anxious I have always been, frankly and generously, to do the fullest and amplest justice to the claims of others.

I am, Sir, &c.,

E. P. CHARLESWORTH, M.D.,

Senior Physician of the Lincoln Asylum.

Lincoln, Jan. 1851.

From the 'LANCET,' *Feb.* 22, 1851.

DISUSE OF INSTRUMENTS OF RESTRAINT IN LUNACY. —THE CLAIMS OF MR R. GARDINER HILL.

[*Letter from Mr R. Gardiner Hill.*]

" SUO SIBI GLADIO HUNC JUGULO."

TO THE EDITOR OF THE 'LANCET.'

SIR,—Truth is always consistent with itself. It is very remarkable that my *recent* opponents, in their letters, do not proceed far in their attacks before they directly contradict their own assertions. Sir E. F. Bromhead set out with stating that "no one could exclusively claim the merit" of the disuse of instrumental restraint, and concluded by asserting that it was Mr Hill who had "the courage to broach the original and invaluable idea that the use of instruments might be WHOLLY dispensed with."

Another equally unexpected opponent now steps forward, in the person of Mr Pierce, a Governor of the Asylum of twenty years' standing, who, of course, is well acquainted with all the proceedings connected with the Asylum, and therefore, if he makes an incorrect assertion, it can scarcely be deemed either accidental or undesigned. Let us therefore briefly examine his letter. He commences with stating that I have " brought forward his name, with that of others, in support of my *recent* claim to be the author and originator of non-restraint." My claim is not a *recent* claim; it was made when the event took place. In June, 1838 (before Sir Edward F. Bromhead, Bart., President of the Mechanics' Institution, and Vice-President of the Lincoln Asylum, who moved a formal vote of thanks to me for it), I delivered a lecture at the Mechanics' Institution at Lincoln, wherein the claim was decisively made, and as decisively proved by reference to the documents and reports of the Asylum, to some of which the name of W. M. Pierce was attached. No other use has been made of his name. This lecture was published in 1839, within two years from the time when I conceived the idea and introduced the system ; from this lecture Mr Pierce quotes a passage, and therefore *knows* that my claim is not *recent*. He then expresses his dissent (!) from this assumption, although his own name is attached to the reports which authorize me to assume it, and says that " Dr Charlesworth is the true author and originator of the non-restraint system." I might here oppose the testimony of Sir E. F. Bromhead, a governor of equal if not longer standing than Mr Pierce, who says that " no one can exclusively claim the merit;" and then, that it was Mr Hill

who " broached the invaluable idea." But I will ask Mr
Pierce to point out one single passage in the records of the
institution which asserts that Dr Charlesworth is the author
and originator of non-restraint. I will ask him, did Dr
Charlesworth himself ever claim to have originated it ?
Where is the evidence that Dr Charlesworth " avowedly
insisted on the abolition of restraint at the Lincoln Asylum,"
previous to my announcing my belief in the possibility and
practicability of it ? Where is one single proof of all these
assertions ?

But, " the exceptional cases " (of restraint) " diminished
with an accelerated rapidity under my predecessor," and " had
he continued a little longer in office, the inevitable result of
Dr Charlesworth's experiments must have been attained
before my appointment." That the total abolition of restraint
was the inevitable result of Dr Charlesworth's experiments
I deny; it was not contemplated; improved instruments
were actually ordered by the Board within less than a year
previous to my appointment, and when I announced the
doctrine of total abolition, it was received at first with
astonishment and incredulity; it was stigmatised as the
raving of a monomaniac, as a dangerous hallucination, and
finally, as a practical breaking of the sixth commandent, by
rashly exposing the lives of the attendants. How far this
result was likely to be attained under my predecessor he
himself will perhaps be esteemed the best judge. Let us
hear, then, what he says: " Restraint forms the very basis
and principle on which the sound treatment of lunatics is
founded. The judicious and appropriate adaptation of the
various modifications of this powerful means to the peculiarities of each case of insanity, comprises a large portion of the
curative regimen of the scientific and rational practitioner;
in his hands it is a remedial agent of the very first importance,
and it appears to me that it is about as likely to be dispensed
with, in the cure of mental diseases, as that the various

articles of the materia medica will be altogether dispensed with in the cure of the bodily."—(Mr Hadwen's letter to the 'Times,' Jan. 25, 1841.) He further says, that "Mr Hill's curious and heterodox opinion, that 'restraint is never necessary, never justifiable, but always injurious in all cases of lunacy whatever,' is more remarkable for its rashness even than its boldness."—(Mr Hadwen's letter to the 'Lancet,' Oct. 1, 1840).

My predecessor, therefore, declares the inevitable result *unattainable;* Mr Pierce declares, that it must have been attained had Mr Hadwen remained a little longer. Let us further see at what period the number of cases of restraint diminished with *most accelerated rapidity.* Take the two years and a half previous to my appointment, and the two years and a half subsequently. In the two years and a half previous to my appointment, there were 186 patients under treatment, of which 84 were restrained for a period of 20, 218$\frac{1}{2}$ hours; in the two years and a half subsequent to my appointment there were 162 patients treated, and 23 were restrained for 1,608 hours. Then, having carefully compared the results of the existing mode of treatment, and having witnessed the agony of one especially who died under the gripe of the iron handcuffs, I came to the conclusion that instrumental restraint was altogether unnecessary and injurious. I announced this opinion to Dr Charlesworth and the Governors; as Mr Pierce truly says, " I declared myself competent to cope with any case whatever," and I acted upon this determination ever after.

Mr Pierce allows that I have indeed "the justly-earned merit of being the first to conjecture a result, which my own subsequent failure proved to be premature, and which Dr Charlesworth was too cautious and philosophic to assume on inadequate induction." But I thought that " Dr Charlesworth was the true author and originator of the non-restraint system." Oh, no! he was "too cautious and philosophic to assume such a result on inadequate induction." Now for the alleged failure: "In April, 1840, a patient was instrumentally restrained for about eighteen hours, but that was through circumstances solely imputable to a disorganised state of the staff of attendants, and not to any failure in the system when carried out in the manner laid down in my Lecture delivered on June 1st, 1838, and published in April, 1839."—(See my letter to the 'Lancet' of November 20, 1842.) In fact, the opposition against me and my system at this period was so violent that I had no resource left but to resign my principles or my appointment. I chose, at every personal sacrifice, the latter alternative.

I know of no reason why my extracts should be distasteful to Mr Pierce, except it be that they prove the justness of my claims. I cannot, however, forbear giving you a few more.

From the eleventh Annual Report of the Lincoln Asylum, April, 1835 :—" A further review of the instruments of restraint has reduced them to four simple methods. * * * The object of restraint is not punishment, but security."

This statement was made only three months previous to my appointment, and is an evident proof that the abolition of restraint was not then contemplated.

Dr Granville, in his 'Spas of England, Midland Division,' p. 87, says—" In speaking of a true and full execution of the plan of not coercing patients, applied to a large lunatic Asylum, in all cases of mental disturbance, no matter of what nature or degree, one is bound to defer the palm of originality and perseverance to Mr Hill, whose work on the subject has probably led the way to a totally new era in the management of insane persons. It is Mr Hill who has the merit of having proposed and undertaken the execution of a method which entails a prodigious increase of labour and responsibility on the medical attendants, and consequently (in the case of the Lincoln Asylum) on himself ; a labour and responsibility, indeed, in which the whole intrinsic value of the system consists."

We come now to Dr Granville's interview with Dr Charlesworth; and here we arrive at those unbiassed sentiments, which, up to the present period, I have always had reason to believe that the doctor entertained. " After a first introduction to the senior physician of the Asylum," says Dr Granville, " he soon put me at my ease by conversing freely and unreservedly on the subject which engrossed my attention at the time, and by frankly avowing himself the staunchest advocate of the plan, *as well as of the originator of it.*"—Id. p. 89.

I could add a score of such extracts, but I prefer concluding with the present one, hoping that Dr Charlesworth will long continue to " avow himself the staunchest advocate of the plan, as well as of the originator of it."

I have the honour to be

Your faithful and obliged servant,

ROBERT GARDINER HILL.

Lincoln, Feb. 3, 1851.

P.S. The reduction of restraints by Mr Hadwen, my predecessor, stated by me (in the extract so " carefully gleaned out " by Mr Pierce, " without reference to context, or the circumstances under which they occurred "), to be in the proportion of seven to one, is not the *average* reduction made by him. It was formed by taking the *highest* number under restraint in one day by Mr Marston (Mr Hadwen's predecessor), and the *lowest* number in one day by Mr Hadwen. The *average* is as follows (see Tables at the end of my Lecture):—1,060 hours per month for the last twelve months of Mr Marston; and 334 hours under Mr Hadwen. The *average* proportion, therefore, was only three to one, instead of seven to one. It should be remembered that the paragraph was written in self-defence, at a time when I, as the originator of the new system of non-restraint, was the object of incessant attacks on all sides.

[*Letter from the Rev. Mr Daniel.*]

Sir,—For the last three weeks I have been told that Dr Charlesworth was about to write a letter to the Lancet, and this formidable letter was held *in terrorem* over the heads of Mr Hill's committee; but lo! it all proves to have been the mountain in labour :—

" Parturiunt montes; nascitur ridiculus mus!" That letter, nevertheless, puny as it is, is remarkable for two things—its ambiguity, and its insinuations. The words reported in the *Eastern Counties Herald* to have been uttered by Dr Charlesworth, at Hull, are these : " The *real* honour of first introducing the system [of non-restraint] belongs to Mr Hill." This is nothing more than what he has said and written before. I remember well the doctor's stating the same fact to me, when he did me the honour to accompany me over a portion of the Lincoln Asylum, during the illness of the house-surgeon, in the summer of 1838. But Dr Charlesworth, in his short and ambiguous reply, says, that he " *doubts* (!) his having expressed himself in these exact terms." Does he remember the exact terms in which he expressed himself to Dr Granville ? If he himself were the originator of the system, would he thus speak ? would the real author of any discovery " doubt " whether he had or had not attributed it to another ? Would he not say at once, not ambiguously, but boldly and unhesitatingly, " The discovery is mine, I am the author of the system ?" And would he not appeal to the records and documents in proof of his assertion ? This is what Mr Hill did in 1839, when he published his lecture on " The Total Abolition of Restraint in the Treatment of the Insane."

It is, however, a matter of no consequence to the arguments whether Dr Charlesworth did or did not " express himself in these exact terms " at the dinner at Hull; there is abundant evidence without it. The abolition of restraint in the Lincoln Asylum, by Mr R. Gardiner Hill, in accordance with his own "bold conception" of its practicability previously announced, *is an established historic fact, which cannot be controverted.* Of this fact there can be no room for *doubt* in the mind of Dr Charlesworth; but as he states in his letter that he " certainly did not contemplate the conclusion which Mr Hill has drawn " from his words, he thereby *insinuates* what I think he will find some difficulty in *proving* —viz. that " the real honour of first introducing the system " *does not* "belong to Mr Hill," and of course that it *does belong* to himself. If this be his meaning, *let him openly avow it.* It would appear, from his own letter, that he is " frankly and generously disposed to do the fullest and amplest justice to the claims of others." I therefore, as Secretary to Mr Hill's committee, do hereby challenge this " frank and generous " man to come forward boldly and manfully, and give a direct answer, without " doubt" or equivocation, to the following questions :—Was it *you* or was it *Mr Hill,* who " *conceived* " and broached the original and invaluable idea, that the use of instruments might be *wholly* dispensed with." Did *you* ever claim this " invaluable idea " as *your own?* I further challenge Dr Charlesworth to state " frankly," (we do not want " *generosity,*" we only want *truth*), in what Report or document of the Asylum the merit of originating the non-restraint or total-abolition system is given to him? —or even to point out a single passage, in any of the Reports, to that effect? The very position of Dr Charlesworth with respect to the Asylum of itself proves that he *could not* originate such a system, nor carry it out if he had. " The responsibility on the point of personal safety could not but rest with the resident officer;" and Dr Charlesworth was only one of the three visiting physicians *in rotation, i. e., for four months out of the twelve.* The House-Surgeon was the resident medical superintendent. The reports of the Asylum are *public documents;* and therein I find Dr Charlesworth's name affixed, as Chairman of the Board of Governors, to the Report which assigns that merit to Mr Hill.

I would beg to observe, in conclusion, that Mr Hill's claims do not in the least derogate from the true merit of Dr Charleswoth, nor afford any just ground of jealousy. His praiseworthy exertions in the amelioration of the condition of the insane have never been denied. I am only astounded that after the repeated testimony which he has himself borne to the fact of Mr Hill's being the author of the non-coercive system, he should now, when a testimonial is proposed to that gentleman, attempt to cast a " *doubt* " upon the fact. The doctor may rest fully assured that *his* popularity, notwithstanding the proposed testimonial to Mr Hill, will still *cleave* unto him as long as he lives.

I am, Sir, yours faithfully,

JOHN DANIEL.

East Ardsley Parsonage, Wakefield,
 Feb. 1, 1851.

[From the ' LANCET,' March 1, 1851.]

DISUSE OF INSTRUMENTS OF RESTRAINT IN THE TREATMENT OF LUNACY.—THE CLAIMS OF MR R. GARDINER HILL.

TO THE EDITOR OF THE ' LANCET.'

Sir,—Dr Charlesworth " doubts" his having used the exact words reported in the *Eastern Counties Herald.* Can he doubt the exact words reported in the *Lancet?* I give you them verbatim: [The *Lancet,* August 24, 1850, pp. 247, 248.] " At the dinner which terminated this agreeable *réunion,* about 100 members of the profession sat down together, with several eminent inhabitants of the town of

Hull. In the course of the evening, Dr Conolly paid a handsome tribute to the labours of Dr Charlesworth, in having, previously to his own exertions, promulgated the system of dispensing with unnecessary restraint in the treatment of the insane; and Dr Charlesworth honourably testified that " the real honour belonged to Mr Hill, of the Lincoln Asylum."

If this be not final and decisive, Mr Editor, why, then, I can only say that men will not be convinced, " though one rose from the dead."

I am, Sir, yours, faithfully,

East Ardley Parsonage,   JOHN DANIEL.
Wakefield, Feb. 24, 1851.

*** Mr Daniel is correct in his quotation; it occurs in our report of the Eighteenth Anniversary Meeting of the Provincial Medical and Surgical Association of Hull, Aug. 6, 1850; and a similar statement found a place in the *Provincial Medical Journal,* which reported the proceedings at the same anniversary.—ED. L.

TO THE EDITOR OF THE ' LANCET.'

Sir,—This affair may now be safely left to the penetration of a very shrewd profession, and to a short parallel.

When Columbus approached the end of his great adventure, he sent a mariner aloft to look out. That mariner saw land, or thought that he saw it, and at the land they shortly arrived. He did his duty manfully, looked out well, and had never flinched, nor taken part with the mutinous crew, but I never heard that he claimed to be the originator of the discovery.

Mr Hill's just claims have never been questioned by any one, and least of all by the real originator of the system.

Your readers will not expect that any notice should be

Q 2

taken of the unbecoming and rude effusion which accompanies Mr Hill's letter.

I am, Sir, your obedient servant,

W. M. PIERCE.

West Ashby, Feb. 25, 1851.

It may not be amiss to insert here the following animadversions on this letter by the Rev. John Daniel, extracted principally from his speech at the Presentation dinner :—

" Mr Pierce leaves ' this affair to the penetration of a very shrewd profession, and to a short parallel.'

" As I believe theprofession to be not only ' *very shrewd,* but also *fair and impartial judges of evidence,* I leave the case in their hands with the greatest satisfaction.

" Had Mr Pierce compared Mr Gardiner Hill to the pilot, who, in the midst of an apparently shoreless ocean, confidently anticipated that land was near, and steered the vessel safe into the harbour, his ' short parallel' would have held good.

" But ' Mr Hill's just claims' (viz. : that he was the originator of the system of the total abolition of restraint,) ' have never been questioned by any one !'—(Then I say they are unquestionably true.)—' Least of all by the real originator of the system !' Is this passage intelligible, or consistent with common sense ?—Let me see if I can find a ' parallel' to it :—

> ' If the man what turnips cries,
> Cries not when his father dies ;
> 'Tis a proof that he would rather
> Have a turnip than his father !'

" There is as much logic in the one sentence as in the other.

" The concluding sentence is a master-piece of ingenuity and condescension ! ' Your readers will not expect that any notice should be taken of the unbecoming and rude effusion which accompanies that letter !'

" There are some men, who, though exquisitely sensitive to the touch themselves, are utterly regardless of the feelings of others. It was, no doubt, quite ' becoming' in Mr Pierce to call Mr Hill ' an agent in an experiment,' ' a mariner sent up aloft to look out,'—and to tell him that ' Dr Charlesworth could have done very well without him ;'—I say, all this was quite ' becoming' in Mr Pierce ;—but the moment he is required to *prove* his assertions, this, *because it affects himself,* is ' unbecoming and rude.'

" One cannot but be struck with the utter absence of evidence, or of any attempt at evidence, in support of the reckless assertions made by Mr Pierce, and allowed by Dr Charlesworth ! But now, in conclusion, I have a serious and important question to ask :—Which of them will compensate Mr Hill for the injury they have done him ? I know that he has been put to a very great—I may ·say— an enormous expense, to defend his just claims :—I know, moreover, that many persons residing at a distance from Lincoln, who had not access to the evidence in Mr Hill's favour, were prevented from subscribing by these unjust statements. I ask, then, who will compensate Mr Hill for the injury done to him ?—It is a part of Christian conduct, not only to *forgive* others, but also (which is a far harder task,) to be ' ready to make restitution and satisfaction, to the uttermost of our power, for all injuries and wrongs *done by us to any other.*'

" Let Mr Pierce remember this, and he will draw no more ' short parallels.' "

To the President, Vice-President, and Governors of the Lincoln Lunatic Asylum.

My Lords, Ladies, and Gentlemen,—I have great pleasure in having permission to publish the following important correspondence between Charles Ward, Esq., Mayor of Lincoln, Chairman of Mr Hill's Committee, the Rev. John

Daniel, Vicar of East Ardsley, near Wakefield, one of the Secretaries, and Archibald Robertson, Esq., M.D., F.R.S., Fellow of the Royal College of Physicians of Edinburgh, *a Vice-President of the Provincial Medical and Surgical Association*, and Physician to the General Infirmary, Northampton.

"Northampton, January 6, 1851.

" Sir,—I have the honour to enclose a post-office order for a guinea, being my mite towards the testimonial proposed to be presented to that highly meritorious gentleman, Mr R. G. Hill, the originator of the system of " non-restraint" in the treatment of the insane.

" The world at large, and the friends of humanity in particular, owe a debt of gratitude to that gentleman : and I hope the proposed testimonial will be something worthy of the man, and of the occasion.

"I am, Sir, your faithful humble servant,

"A. ROBERTSON, M.D., F.R.S.

" To the Rev. John Daniel, East Ardsley."

"Northampton, Feb. 24, 1851.

" Sir,—I am astonished to find, from a printed circular received this morning, bearing your signature, that a question has arisen as to the rightful claim of Mr Robert Gardiner Hill to be the originator of the humane system of ' non-restraint' in the treatment of lunacy.

"I can only say, that, at the Annual Meeting of the Provincial Medical Association, held at Hull in August last, the claim of Mr R. G. Hill to that discovery (for it *is* a discovery, and a most important one) was gracefully conceded to Mr Hill by Dr Conolly, of Hanwell,—who, to say the very least, is a highly competent judge; and that Mr Hill's claim, and the merit due to it, were ratified by the unanimous assent and approval of that numerous meeting.

" I cannot help, as a subscriber to Mr Hill's testimonial, placing that fact before you; as it possibly may not be known to yourself and the other gentlemen forming the committee.

"I have the honour to be, Sir,

"Your faithful humble servant,

"A. ROBERTSON, M.D., F.R.S.

"To Charles Ward, Esq., Mayor of Lincoln."

"Lincoln, Feb. 25, 1851.

"Sir,—I beg to acknowlege the receipt of your communication of yesterday, upon the subject of the testimonial to Mr R. Gardiner Hill, for originating the system of 'nonrestraint' in the treatment of lunatics. I feel it my duty to inform you that the *cause* of the *publication* of the *circular* and *advertisement* having *my* signature attached, arises from the fact that Mr Pierce has addressed the public, *claiming* the honour of *originality* for Dr Charlesworth. The Committee having the charge of Mr Hill's claims, after perusing the documentary *evidence* in which Dr C. is *strongly* implicated, have resolved to proceed.

"In your note to me you appear to have a very *distinct* recollection of what passed at the Annual Meeting of the Provincial Medical Association, held at Hull in August last; at *that* meeting Dr Charlesworth *is reported* to have stated, that the *real honour of first introducing* the system *was due to Mr Hill,* I take the liberty of asking you whether you *recollect* Dr Charlesworth making use of that expression *at the meeting,* which is corroborated and fully borne out by the publication of the proceedings in the *Lancet, Eastern Counties Herald,* &c., and the favour of your reply upon that point will be much appreciated by Mr Hill and his committee.

"I remain, Sir, your obedient servant,

"CHARLES WARD,

"Chairman of the Committee.

"Dr A. Robertson, Northampton."

"P.S. I communicate to you as the Chairman of the Committee, and disclaim all personal interference with Dr Charlesworth, for whom I entertain strong feelings of confidence and respect, and the doctor is my consulting medical physician, when required."

"Lincoln, Feb. 25, 1851.

"Dear Sir,—The Mayor of Lincoln has given me leave to add a few words to his answer to your kind letter received yesterday. Let me inform you, then, that Dr Charlesworth voluntarily called upon Mr Hill, told him that he had received a letter from Dr Conolly, who meant to give the credit of 'non-restraint' to Lincoln, and that he (Dr Charlesworth) wished to give credit where credit was due, and therefore requested Mr Hill to accompany him to Hull, which he did accordingly—with what result you know. Mr Hill's claims are corroborated by a series of incontrovertible evidence, throughout a period of twelve or thirteen years, and were never called into question here until the proposal of this testimonial, when Mr Pierce attempted to claim the thing for his friend Dr Charlesworth. But I happen to have Dr Charlesworth's sign-manual to the contrary; his handwriting appears in the very MSS. letters to *the Lancet*, in which Mr Hill makes his strongest assertion of his claim in answer to various opponents of the system.

"Moreover, when Dr Charlesworth did me the honour to accompany me over a portion of the Asylum, in 1838, he told me that the entire absence of restraint which I then observed, was owing to the indefatigable labours of Mr Hill.

"These MSS. will be published, if necessary.

"Believe me, dear Sir, yours faithfully,

"JOHN DANIEL.

"A. Robertson, Esq., M.D."

"Northampton, March 7, 1851.

"Sir,—I am very sorry that a succession of very pressing professional occupations has prevented me from sooner replying to your letter of the 25th of February.

"In that letter you state that 'Mr Pierce has addressed the public, claiming the honour of *originality* for Dr Charlesworth' as to the discovery and first practice of the 'non-restraint' system in the treatment of lunatics. You go on to ask whether I 'recollect Dr Charlesworth making use of the expression at the meeting of the Provincial Medical Association, held at Hull in August last, that the '*real honour of first introducing* the system *was due to Mr Hill*'?

"When thus appealed to, I have no hesitation in saying that I have a very distinct recollection of the above expressions having been made use of by Dr Charlesworth, or words to that effect. The information made the greater impression upon me, as it was perfectly new to *me*; so vague and imperfect was my knowledge as to the first discovery and practice of the 'non-restraint' system, prior to the Hull meeting, that I had thought the merit of it belonged to Dr Conolly of Hanwell. Acting upon this thought, I had, very shortly before the Hull meeting, subscribed my mite towards a testimonial to Dr Conolly: which had been suggested at a meeting in London, presided over by Lord Ashley. But when I heard, at the Hull meeting, the credit of having really originated the 'non-restraint' system frankly and gracefully declined by Dr Conolly on the one hand, and by Dr Charlesworth on the other, and *by both* unhesitatingly ascribed to Mr R. G. Hill, I could not for a moment doubt that the latter gentleman had the honour and the high merit of having originated this vast improvement in the treatment of lunacy.

"Although I happened to sit very near to Dr Conolly, Dr Charlesworth, and Mr Hill, at the Hull meeting, and was not likely to hear imperfectly what was said on the occasion,

I have been anxious to test the accuracy of my recollection of their words by a reference to the report contained in the *Provincial Medical and Surgical Journal* I enclose an extract from the report, and by it you will perceive that there is no mistake in what (I thought and believed) I had distinctly heard.

    " I have the honour to be, Sir,

        " Your faithful and humble Servant,

            " A. ROBERTSON, M.D.

" To Charles Ward, Esq., Mayor of Lincoln."

            " Northampton, March 8th, 1851.

    " Dear Sir,—I received your letter of the 25th of February, and I am sorry that I have been thus tardy in acknowledging it. My silence has been owing to a temporary pressure of occupation.

    " I am greatly concerned to hear that an attempt has been set on foot to rob Mr R. G. Hill of the honour, so justly his due, of PRIORITY in the invention and practical application of the ' non-restraint' system to the treatment of insanity. I shall be still more concerned if it should turn out, which I am slow to believe, that Dr Charlesworth has lent any countenance to such attempt. However, I have the satisfaction of knowing that the matter is in highly competent hands; and that you, and the other gentlemen of committee, will see thorough justice done to Mr Hill.

    " I wrote yesterday to the Mayor of Lincoln, in answer to his letter of the 25th ult. addressed to me, in which he requested to know if I had a DISTINCT recollection of what fell from Dr Charlesworth at the Hull meeting. I have answered his letter at some length, and have appended an extract from the speeches at the Hull meeting, as reported in our recognised organ, the *Provincial Medical and Surgical Journal.* I need not speak of the contents of my letter at more length: as I take it for granted it will be laid, by the Mayor, before yourself and the other members of Mr Hill's Committee.

"I am no partisan in this matter, but an unbiassed witness. I have every friendly disposition, both to Dr Charlesworth and Mr Hill, as respected members of the same professson with myself; and would gladly do a kindness to either of them. '*Sed magis amica veritas.*' When appealed to, as I have been, in this business, I feel that I have nothing to consider but the cause of truth. For this reason I have spoken openly and conclusively in favour of Mr Hill's priority of claim. You are free to make any use of this letter you may think proper.

"Believe me to be, dear Sir, with great respect,
"Yours faithfully,
"A. ROBERTSON, M.D.
"Rev. J. Daniel, East Ardsley, Wakefield."

Mr R. Gardiner Hill and his friends have now laid before you and the public a series of evidence which must be conclusive in support of his claim to be the originator of the "non-restraint" system.

I have the honour to be,
My Lords, Ladies, and Gentlemen,
Your faithful and obedient Servant,
RICHARD SUTTON HARVEY,
A Governor of the Lincoln Lunatic Asylum.
Lincoln, March 12th, 1851.

From the 'LANCET' *March* 15, 1851.
DISUSE OF INSTRUMENTAL RESTRAINT IN THE
TREATMENT OF THE INSANE.—THE CLAIMS
OF MR R. GARDINER HILL.

TO THE EDITOR OF THE 'LANCET.'

Sir,—This question cannot rest upon the accuracy or interpretation of expressions used at the Provincial Association at Hull. The report in the *Provincial Medical and Surgical Journal'* to which you make a reference in your last number, did not give entire satisfaction, as will appear in the subjoined letter, Oct. 25th, 1850.

I am, Sir your obedient Servant,

E. P. CHARLESWORTH.

Lincoln, March, 3, 1851.

(Copy.)

TO THE EDITOR OF THE 'PROVINCIAL MEDICAL AND SURGICAL
JOURNAL.'

Sir,—Will you allow me to correct an error in the report of my speech at Hull, which appears in your journal of August 21st? You therein report thus of my observations:—'He (Mr Hill) was bound to acknowledge that the system (of non-restraint) did, *to some extent,* (!) originate with himself.' Now the words 'to some extent,' were never uttered by me, and seem to throw a doubt upon my being, as the records of the Lincoln Asylum indisputably and indelibly prove me to be, the sole author and originator of the total abolition or non-restraint system in the treatment of lunatics.

I shall be obliged to you to insert this my correction of your statement. To Dr Conolly belongs the merit of adopting and carrying out this system, in an institution eight times as large as that of Lincoln, and I trust the public testimonial which is about to be presented to that gentleman will be worthy of the great services which he has rendered to mankind. But as he himself frankly and honourably avowed, and as from my own knowledge of him I am sure he will again at any time avow, he was not the author of that system. The merit of that, be it more or less, is not one which, as your leading article of September 4th would seem to imply, *may* be justly due to me, but one which no

one else çan claim, and of which I shall not allow any
one to rob me.

I am, Sir, your obedient Servant,

ROBERT GARDINER HILL.

[The words in '*italics*' are so printed in the original.]

To the President, Vice-Presidents, and Governors of the
Lincoln Asylum.

My Lords, Ladies, and Gentlemen,—I make no apology for
bringing before your notice the 21st Report of the Asylum,
drawn up by Sir Edward Ff. Bromhead, Bart., and the
auditors, because it appears with my name appended to it.*
Of the Report itself I have little to say, excepting as regards
the concluding paragraph. With respect to the annexed
" Minutes," as they are called, it appears to me that the main
object in appending them, in the form in which they are got
up, is to make a covert attack upon the rightful claims of
Mr R. Gardiner Hill to be the originator of " non-restraint "
or " total abolition."†

I will first speak of this paragraph of the Report itself,
and then of the annexed " Minutes."

The 21st Report concludes with these words:—" The

---

* " The 21st Annual Report, with the proceedings of the Lincoln Lunatic
Asylum annexed to it, and published in 1845, professedly bears my signature,
which signature I never gave. I occupied the chair but a very short time, and did
not conduct the business of the meeting to a conclusion, being early called away.
During my stay, neither the ' *Report* ' nor the ' proceedings' were produced to the
board in my presence ; and *to this day the draft minutes of that meeting remain
unsigned.*"—Speech of R. S. Harvey, Esq., at the Presentation dinner.

† "I leave you to judge my astonishment when I tell you that, on inquiry,
Messrs W. & B. Brooke informed me that they printed those 'proceedings,' &c.,
for Dr Charlesworth, and that they were paid for by him *in his private account.*
From the Asylum minutes I learned that Dr Charlesworth offered to supply the
Governors ' gratuitously ' with as many copies of the ' proceedings ' as might be
wanted, to be annexed to the annual Report. On the board accepting them, they
were stitched up with the 21st Report, and allowed to be circulated as an Asylum
document."—Idem.

Governors will find appended to the present statement, an abstract of the successive proceedings in this house towards the system of abolishing mechanical restraint; shewing that that system was the unexpected result of gradual progressive improvement and experience, and not the result of any theory or attempt at effect."

As this may at first sight appear contrary to the observations of Sir E. Ff. Bromhead, Bart., on "the soundness of the non-restraint *theory*," when, as President of the Mechanics' Institution, he moved a formal vote of thanks to Mr Hill, for his Lecture "on the total abolition of restraint," I shall beg to offer the following explanations :—The new doctrine was stigmatized as "the raving of a theoretic visionary," &c. &c., whereas Mr Hill "expressed his *belief, founded on experience*" in the Lincoln Asylum, "that it might be possible to conduct an institution for the treatment of the insane, without having recourse to the employment of any instrument of restraint whatever."[*] Here is the origin of the "*sound theory*," which was *thenceforward* adopted in practice by Mr Hill, and a very different thing it is from "the raving of a *theoretic* visionary," or "*any attempt at effect*," which the Report very properly stigmatizes.

That it was, nevertheless, a "*theory*," and a "*sound*" one, too,[†] we have not only the testimony of Sir E. Ff. Bromhead, but that of Dr Charlesworth also. The *original preface* to Mr Hill's lecture (which differs *materially* from the one published) was submitted by Mr Hill to Dr Charlesworth for his approval, and in the sentence "the *theory* verified by the practice," the words "verified by the practice" are in Dr Charlesworth's handwriting. The original preface, and the Doctor's alterations, can be seen by any one who will

---

[*] Report, 1837.

[†] "For it *is* a discovery, and a most important one."—Dr A. Robertson, F.R.S., Northampton.

take the trouble to examine them. They will most probably be published before long.*

As regards the "minutes," which are appended to the Report, this is apparent: that the resolution of 1843,† which is so prominently brought forth in capital letters, instead of being described as *the result of Mr Hill's " bold conception," and subsequent verification of it*, which it truly is, is introduced as the result of " the progessive proceedings under which the total abolition of instrumental restraint was introduced and established in the Lincoln Lunatic Asylum." This is unfair and unjust to Mr Hill in the highest possible degree. Mr Hill announced his confident belief in the practicability of this plan to Dr Charlesworth and the Governors, in 1837,— he acted upon it, he carried it out—his complete success approved it—suicides disappeared under it—not one fatal accident occurred—the proportion of recoveries increased— the reputation and the funds of the Asylum rose—its prosperity was enhanced—the number of patients was greatly augmented—and yet the framers of these *" minutes "* now wish to pledge the Governors generally to requite Mr Hill's services, not only with a cool and studied reserve, but even with ingratitude.

To show that I have not used too strong language, I appeal from the *"minutes "* to the review of Mr Hill's Lecture in the

---

* The passage referred to was the following :—"It may be desirable to state here once for all what is due to the Institution, and what I may fairly claim &c." —This passage was omitted by Dr Charlesworth, because, as he observed, " the abolition of restraint belonged to me and *would never be disputed*; it was given to me in the Reports, and therefore the insertion of the passage was merely *fighting with a shadow*." These were Dr Charlesworth's own words to me, as I find from a letter written by me at the time to a friend," and on these grounds it was omitted, unfortunately for myself, as it would have prevented much subsequent disputation and annoyance that was never anticipated.—R. G. H.

† 1843, July 12. At a quarterly board, &c.—Resolved, THAT EVERY IN-STRUMENT OF RESTRAINT IN THIS HOUSE BE FORTHWITH REMOVED FROM THE PREMISES, DESTROYED, OR OTHERWISE DISPOSED OF.

Lincoln Standard of the 15th of May, 1839, written by Sir E. Ff. Bromhead, and revised by Dr Charlesworth..* From that review I make the following extracts :—

"Mr Hill had for some time successfully carried into operation, at our Asylum, the total abolition of all restraint, and all severity, before he presented himself to the public as the deliverer of a Lecture on the subject." * * * * *
"In this Lecture, Mr Hill exhibits a frightful picture of the ancient abuses universally inflicted on the insane, until the benevolent Pinel made an inroad on this domain of cruelty. He *began* what Mr Hill *completed*." * * * * * "At Lincoln the Boards resolutely set about to ameliorate the treatment, and have confirmed the remark, 'were every one to see the whole effects, mediate and immediate, present and remote, even of trifling acts of good or evil, his mind would, on many occasions, be filled with delight or remorse.' *The Governors never expressed a wish for the extinction of restraints ; they never expected it ; not one of them deemed it possible ;*† they did all the good they could in a proper direction, they mitigated evil. They elected an honest, firm, sensible, and benignant medical man as a resident officer ; they placed every possible facility in his way ; and this honest and good man‡ found himself landed triumphantly on an unhoped for territory. He had much to struggle with‖ ;—the character of visionary humanity—the underplot of reluctant servants§,

---

* "The article in the *Standard* was written by Sir E. Ff. Bromhead, and revised by Dr Charlesworth."—Letter from Mr R. G. Hill. to the Rev. J. Daniel, Deene Rectory, Wandsford, May 31st, 1839.

† "He" (Mr Hill) "has diligently applied all the means of amelioration placed at his disposal, and in so doing has *conceived and effected results* honourable to himself, and *beyond the hopes of the Board. The practice of restraint and coercion has disappeared under his management*."—Dr Charlesworth.

‡ Whom they now wish to deprive of his hard-earned laurels.

‖ But not, until now, with falsehood and ingratitude.

§ Which, on one occasion, viz., in April, 1840, occasioned a departure of eighteen hours from the system (see Report, 1841).

who found every step in his progress a trespass on their own repose ; and it may be considered most fortunate for mankind that no unlucky *apropos* fatal accident blasted the plan for ever."

If then, " the Governors never expressed a wish for the extinction of restraints "—if " they never expected it "—and " not one of them deemed it possible "—how can Mr Hill be " an agent in an experiment to which he has no claim whatever "! Shame! Shame! I blush that such a sentence should proceed from a governor of the Asylum of twenty years standing. That Mr Hill was " an agent " in such an experiment, is just as true as that the Duke of Wellington was an agent in an experiment made by the British Nation on the balance of power in Europe:—*i. e.* he was the agent by whose bold and decisive genius the plan of battle was devised, and by whose cool and determined courage and perseverance, *the victory was achieved.*

The framers of the minutes, in speaking of the disuse of seclusion, quote the eighteenth report thus.—" This great improvement had been actually in practice, *even during a period of eighteen months in succession,* in this institution ; but the present house-surgeon (Mr Smith), had the firmness formally to disavow, on principle, seclusion altogether, as a means of control." Why was the following remarkable sentence omitted, which was published in 1842, suppressed in these annexed minutes of 1845, but re-appears in 1847 ? " Any previous intervals of disuse, no more detract from his claim in this case, than the occasional absence of instrumental restraint can be considered derogating from the formal abolition of instruments in this house," *i. e.* Mr Smith is fairly and justly entitled to the formal abolition of seclusion as a means of control, and Mr Hill is fairly and justly entitled to the formal abolition of instrumental restraint in this house.—' *Leave this out,*' say the framers of the

R

minutes; *if inserted it will tell in favour of Mr Hill's claims.*"*

Lastly, those minutes are prefaced with the introduction, being chiefly appendix (A) of Mr R. G. Hill's publication on the " Total Abolition of Personal Restraint in the Treatment of the Insane ;" leaving it to be inferred that Mr Hill assents to the statement that " that system was the unexpected result of gradual and progressive experience, and not of any theory "—for as to " attempt at effect "—the idea is too contemptible to entertain for a moment.

Here, again, is unfairness to Mr Hill, whose publication bears date 1839, and, consequently, *cannot* have anything to do with the last five years of the Minutes, and who " certainly never contemplated the inference " which the framers of those minutes " drew from " that appendix (A).

But what was the object of this " *suppressio veri* " in the " annexed minutes,"† the disengenuous heading, and the statement that the abolition of restraint was, in any sense, the result of progressive improvement and not of any theory? What was the object of all this ? I think I can explain it : —It was that some bold man might hereafter declare Dr Charlesworth " the true author and originator of 'non-restraint.' " That some such latent design was intended becomes every day more apparent : for it is whispered in Lincoln that Mr Pearce is following in the wake of Mr Hill's friends, by proposing a subscription testimonial for Dr Charlesworth. Had not Mr Pierce better " busy himself " first in *proving* Dr Charlesworth the author of the

---

* By the Board Minutes for 1842, and 1845, Sir E. Ff. Bromhead and the auditors were requested to prepare the annual reports for those years; will they give the governors a reason for the omission of this part of the report of 1842, in *what are called* the annexed minutes of 1845.

† Which were stitched up with the Annual Report for 1845, " printed and circulated by the Auditors and Dr Charlesworth."

non-restraint system, rather than in endeavouring to obtain for him a testimonial on grounds which Dr Charlesworth himself has repeatedly assigned to Mr Hill ? * It is to the *grand* " DISCOVERY " made by Mr Hill, in 1837, and published by him in 1839, that we are indebted for the resolution of 1843, " THAT EVERY INSTRUMENT OF RESTRAINT IN THIS HOUSE " (*being useless thanks to Mr Hill*) " BE FORTH-WITH REMOVED FROM THE PREMISES, DESTROYED, OR OTHERWISE DISPOSED OF."

> I have the honour to be,
> My Lords, Ladies, and Gentlemen,
> Your faithful and obedient servant,
> RICHARD SUTTON HARVEY,
> A Governor of fourteen years standing.

Lincoln, February 26, 1851.

P.S.—The *incontrovertible* documents referred to as evidence of the truthfulness of his claims by Mr Hill's committee, at its second special meeting, held at the Saracen's Head, on Friday, February 21st, 1851, I have not yet published. *They refer to Mr Hill's claims and implicate Dr Charlesworth alone.*

To the President, Vice-Presidents, and Governors of the Lincoln Lunatic Asylum.

My Lords, Ladies, and Gentlemen,—At the conclusion of my last address to you occurs the following passage:—" It is whispered in Lincoln† that Mr Pierce is following in the wake of Mr Hill's friends, by proposing a subscription testimonial for Dr Charlesworth." In reference to this

---

* " The real honour belonged to Mr Hill, of the Lincoln Asylum." Dr Charlesworth's speech at the dinner of the Provincial Medical and Surgical Association at Hull, August 8, 1850, as reported in the ' LANCET ' of August 24, 1850.

† Mr Diamond's information was, of course, communicated to Mr Hill's committee, and consequently spoken of in Lincoln.

passage I received the following letter from the Rev. W. M. Pierce, M.A.

> "Sea-Bank Cottage, Sutton, near Alford,
> "March 1, 1851.

"Sir,—Your printed letter, addressed to the Governors of the Lincoln Lunatic Asylum, has just reached me; I should not have troubled you with any remark upon it but for your observation, "that I am proposing a subscription testimonial to Dr Charlesworth." I think I am fairly entitled to ask the authority upon which you have ventured such an assertion, and I do ask it.

"At the same time, I declare that there is not the *slightest truth* nor *the shadow of truth* in the statement you have presumed to make, and I, therefore, call upon you to give it a positive contradiction, at least to the same extent you have circulated the falsehood itself.

> "I am, Sir, your obedient servant,
> "W. M. PIERCE.

"To R. S. Harvey, Esq."

Without retracting one atom of the statement I have made; without being under any necessity of contradicting what Mr Pierce, with as much elegance as good humour, terms, "a falsehood," not having *the slightest truth,* or the *shadow of truth* in it, I shall entreat your attention for one moment to the subjoined letters.

> "Lincoln, March 5th, 1851.

"Dear Sir,—I beg to call your attention to the communication you made me respecting Sir A. Morrison having sent Mr Pierce five guineas on behalf of Dr Charlesworth; will you grant me permission to make use of your information?

> "I am, dear Sir, yours faithfully,
> "RICHARD SUTTON HARVEY.

"Hugh W. Diamond, Esq., Surrey County Asylum."

" Surrey County Lunatic Asylum, near Wandsworth,
" March 6th, 1851.

" My dear Sir,—In reply to your enquiries, I beg to assure you that what I stated to you in my letter of the 19th of February, is perfectly correct. After the appearance of Mr Pierce's letter in the 'Lancet,' I spoke to Sir Alexander Morrison on the subject of Mr Hill's testimonial, and he then informed me that he had received a letter from Mr Pierce, and that he had sent him five guineas for Dr Charlesworth.

" I have never myself doubted Mr Hill's claims to be the originator of what is now called the 'non-restraint' system of treatment towards the insane; and I think, that after what has lately appeared, no one else can with fairness do so. I beg you will make whatever use of this letter you may deem necessary, and I can only add that I am very glad to hear you are making such good progress in regard to the subscription.

" I am, dear Sir, very faithfully yours,

" Hugh W. Diamond, F.S.A.

" To R. S. Harvey, Esq."

Hence it appears that *in reply to a letter received from Mr Pierce,* Sir Alexander Morrison sent him five guineas for Dr Charlesworth, although he had previously subscribed to Mr Hill's testimonial; therefore instead of retracting " a falsehood," I have the more pleasing task of verifying by authority the truth of my statement.

I have the honour to be,

My Lords, Ladies, and Gentlemen,

Your faithful and obedient Servant,

Richard Sutton Harvey,

A Governor of the Lincoln Lunatic Asylum.

Lincoln, March 11th, 1851.

To the President, Vice-Presidents, and Governors of the
Lincoln Lunatic Asylum.

My Lords, Ladies, and Gentlemen,—Having taken an active part in the matter of Mr Hill's claims, I am anxious to lay before you such evidence as may be perfectly conclusive with respect to those claims. For this purpose I respectfully invite your attention, first, to the note from Sir E. Ff. Bromhead on his receiving an author's copy of Mr Hill's Lecture, published in 1839. Next, to Sir Edward's letter, addressed to the " Chairman of the Lunatic Asylum, Bodmin," wherein he calls the system then in operation in the Lincoln Lunatic Asylum "his" (Mr Hill's), and him "the author" of it. The next two letters from Mr Hill, addressed to the Editor of the 'Lancet,' in July and November, 1842, demonstrate the fact that Dr Charlesworth then assented to his claim. In the first of these letters Mr Hill challenges his anonymous opponents to give their real names, and refers to his own " prominent position as the originator of the total abolition of instrumental restraint in lunacy." This letter was submitted to Dr Charlesworth for his inspection previous to publication, and the doctor identifies himself with its contents by the introduction of the word " self" before protection, as indicating still more strongly the personal protection from those acrimonious and anonymous attacks, to which Mr Hill's " prominent position as the originator of total abolition then exposed him." In the second of these letters Mr Hill repeats his claim, and speaks of instrumental restraint having been abolished in the Lincoln Lunatic Asylum, under his superintendance, so early as January, 1837. One single exception is named and accounted for, of which Dr Charlesworth supplies the date, in his own hand-writing. Mr Hill further declares the failure "solely imputable to a disorganized state of the staff of attendants, and not to any failure in the system when carried out in the manner laid down in his Lecture, delivered June 21, 1838, and published in April, 1839." In the next paragragh Mr Hill challenges a pre-claimant to his system, and then congratulates the Editor of the 'Lancet,' the public, and "especially" the insane, upon claimants coming forward to dispute the honour of that invention, which at first was stigmatized with every opprobrious epithet. It is evident, therefore, that in 1842 Dr Charlesworth was cognizant of Mr Hill's claims in both these letters, of his challenge for a pre-claimant to his system, and of his congratulation to the public on the successful issue of his labours. And from all this Mr Hill and his friends were surely justified in supposing that what Dr Charlesworth approved and supported in 1842 he would equally approve and support in 1851.

The proposal of a testimonial to Mr Hill was not in any spirit of opposition or slight to Dr Charlesworth, who was one of the first invited to be on the Committee.

I have the honour to be,
Your faithful and obedient servant,
RICHARD SUTTON HARVEY.

Lincoln, April 3, 1851.

Note from Sir Edward Ff. Bromhead to Mr R. Gardiner Hill, on his receiving an author's copy of his Lecture :

My dear Sir, —You so well know my opinion of your publication and of your asylum exploits, that I need only thank you for the compliment and kindness shown in sending me an author's copy.

Ever truly yours,
E. FF. BROMHEAD.

May, 1839.

Sir Edward Ff. Bromhead's letter, addressed to "the Chairman of the Lunatic Asylum, Bodmin," dated November 6, 1840, will be found in Appendix (B), page 186. Quoted also in Appendix (C).

Rough copies of two letters, written by Mr R. Gardiner Hill, addressed to the Editor of the 'Lancet,' and published July and November, 1842. The words in *italics* are in the handwriting of Dr Charlesworth.

TO THE EDITOR OF THE 'LANCET.'

Sir, — If your correspondents "Exetasticos" and "Quæstor" will favour myself and the public with their real names, I will be happy to reply to their communications through your journal. The acrimonious attacks to which my prominent position as the originator of the total abolition of instrumental restraint in lunacy, have exposed me from its opponents, make it necessary that I should resort to this measure of *self*-protection from irresponsible antagonists.

I am, Sir,

Your obedient and faithful servant,

ROBERT GARDINER HILL.

Lincoln, July 23, 1842.

Sir,—In the number of your journal, to which in your last you have referred me, I find a communication from Dr Finch, claiming as his own, not a total abolition of instrumental restraint in his establishment at Laverstock House, but a per centage of exemption from such means of coercing his patients, I ground the claim, which I have made to the "total abolition of instrumental restraint," upon the fact of its having been abolished in the Lincoln Asylum, under my superintendance, in January, 1837.

It is true that in one single case since the above date, *viz., in April*, 1840, a patient was instrumentally restrained *for eighteen hours,* through circumstances solely imputable to a disorganized state of the staff of attendants, and not to any failure in the system, when carried out in the manner laid down in my Lecture, delivered June 21, 1838, and published in April, 1839. I still wait for a pre-claimant to the system of totally abolishing instrumental restraint in the management of the insane.

And now, Mr Editor, allow me to congratulate yourself and the public, and *especially* the insane, upon the happy turn which the debate upon this subject, occupying so many of your pages, has at length taken. Instead of hearing any longer of the impracticability, the futility, or the absurdity of the system, denominated by its opponents as "Utopian," "speculative," "peculative," &c., &c., you have now in the field combatants for the honour of the invention.

To the President, Vice-Presidents, and Governors of the Lincoln Lunatic Asylum.

My Lords, Ladies, and Gentlemen,—I had hoped to have been spared the necessity of addressing you on a subject relative to myself and my own recognized rights, but the unfair and abusive attacks to which I have been subject, forbid me to remain silent. I am accused by Mr Pierce of being ungrateful to Dr Charlesworth, when, in point of fact, I have on every occasion acknowledged the valuable assistance I received from that gentleman in carrying out my theory of the possibility of the total abolition of restraint, and publicly thanked him for it. Nor do the circulars, in which a testimonial was proposed to me, speak disparagingly of him or his services to the institution, directly or indirectly. They simply assert a matter of fact, proved by the records of the institution, and by a series of evidence from 1837 to the present time, and on that ground propose a testimonial to me.

But what is the present conduct of those very men,

whose testimonies at the time are recorded in indelible
characters to the truth of my claims ? They now attempt to
deny the identical facts which they have themselves attested.

1. Mr Pierce, *e. g.* talks of my "present *pretensions ;*"
and, when speaking of the *general principle* which I announced of the practicability of dispensing with the use
of instruments altogether, he *asserts* that it was a mere
"conjecture," and would willingly represent it as a "barren
speculation !" "Eheu ! quantum mutatis ab illo," Pierce,
who in 1837 attested not only that the "bold conception"
of non-restraint was "due" to me, but that I had, *even
then*, "made a striking advance towards *verifying my
opinion*, by conducting the male (the completed) side of
the house, with but a solitary instance of such restraint,
either by day or by night, during the course of the last
sixteen months, and that applied only for two hours"—
when ?—" during mg absence !" In 1837, then, Mr Pierce
attests that I not only "broached the original and invaluable idea" of non-restraint, but that I had even then
"made a striking advance towards verifying it." And this
report of 1837, be it known to all men, *was written by
Dr Charlesworth*, for he received the thanks of the Board
for drawing it up ; and it was signed by Mr Pierce as
chairman ! And yet this is the man who, ever since the
proposal of a public testimonial to me, has exerted himself
to the utmost of his power to damage the amount of the
testimonial, and has compelled me, by his untrue assertion,*
to defend my claim at an enormous expense, not (as formerly) against anonymous opponents, but against those
very persons whose own previous evidence is at variance
with their present statements !

* Viz.,—That "the true author and originator of non-restraint is Dr Charlesworth ;" whereas Sir E. Ff. Bromhead declares, "the governors never expressed
a wish for the extinction of restraint ; they never expected it, not one of them "—
No ! not even Dr Charlesworth or Mr Pierce—"deemed it possible."

2. Dr Charlesworth, when speaking of the total abolition of restraint, used generally to call it " Hill's system,"
and accordingly assisted me, on 'more than one occasion, to
defend my claim to it against the attacks of various
opponents—for the acrimonious attacks, be it remembered,
were made upon me, not upon Dr Charlesworth; and I, as
the author of the system, defended it. But now, when
Mr Pierce has the *modesty* to contradict both himself and
Dr Charlesworth, and to assert that Dr Charlesworth is the
true author and originator of non-restraint, I am called
ungrateful, because I cannot admit a claim which has no
foundation in truth. Dr Charlesworth *mitigated*, but never
dreamt of *abolishing* restraint. A non-resident visiting
physician, in monthly rotation, *could not* do that, nor be
responsible for the consequence of an order to do it. " The
responsibility could not but rest with the resident officer."
Let the following entries by Dr Charlesworth in the *physician's journal*, speak for themselves :—

" 1840, Oct. 1st. — The House-surgeon (Mr Smith)
having applied to me for special directions as to the sitting-
room in which Miss A. should be placed, I have told him
that such matters must rest with the ability and discretion
of the House-surgeon, who resides on the spot, and will be
guided by the variations which may occur in the cases
placed under his charge."

If Dr Charlesworth, when applied to by the House-
surgeon for special directions, refuses to give them, how
can any House-surgeon be said to carry out Dr Charlesworth's views, or to be a mere " agent in an experiment?"
The simple fact is, that Mr Pierce himself is an " agent in
an experiment,"—and a dishonest one too—to make the
world believe that Dr Charlesworth did what every document connected with the Asylum, and his own public and
deliberate disclaimer, prove that he did not do.

Again, 1841, Jan. 3rd.—" The bold position taken by Mr Hill in his publication on the non-restraint system, assuming the practicability of a total abolition of instrumental restraint, was not less sensible than sound. The present House-surgeon has taken a similar position, as regards the abolition of solitary confinement; and I trust he will succeed in his object, *as Mr Hill has done in his own.*"

(Signed)   " E. P. CHARLESWORTH."

Here Dr Charlesworth bears witness to my *success :* he does not (as Mr Pierce does) use the insulting expression, that I was " an agent in an experiment," " a mariner sent up aloft to look out;" nor does he say with Mr Pierce that I " *failed*" to establish my " conjecture"—(woe unto me if I had!)—but he avers that the position I had taken was not less sensible than sound, and that I had " *succeeded in my object.*" In other words, I carried out my own theory of non-restraint, and demonstrated its practicability.

Why then should Dr Charlesworth " *doubt*" whether or not he bore the same honourable testimony to the truth at Hull, which he had done before ? And when, by the overwhelming evidence of the numbers who heard him, he is driven from this subterfuge, how can he state that " this affair cannot rest upon the accuracy (!) or the interpretation of expressions used at the Provincial Association at Hull ? " What ! cannot this affair depend upon the *accuracy* of his own reported speech ? Cannot his own testimony, even if *accurately reported*, establish the truth of any fact ? Astounding piece of intelligence ! Proh ! pudor ! Proh ! Dii immortales !

Contrast the present conduct of Dr Charlesworth, an *avowed* friend both of myself and my system, with that of the late Dr W. Cookson, long a determined opponent of the non-restraint system. Dr Cookson's recantation of his accusations against " Hill's system," entered by himself in the physician's journal of the Lincoln Asylum, Feb. 24, 1844, and published in the *Lancet* of the 2nd of March following, is a manly and candid avowal of his conviction, which does immortal honour to his memory !

The passage I have quoted above from the physician's journal was entered by Dr Charlesworth in 1841, after my resignation. Mr Pierce, however, says that within the last three months of my office I twice broke down, and was privately remonstrated with by the physician ! This assertion is in accordance with the whole tissue of contradictions which per vade Mr Pierce's letter. How utterly untrue the assertion is that the physician remonstrated with me, let the physicians own entries bear witness :—

1840, April 4.—" C. A., a violent patient, is secluded in her sleeping apartment in the North Gallery, her presence among the other patients being considered unsafe while the taller nurse is engaged in cleaning ; the smaller two nurses not having any control over this patient, and being " afraid of her."

13th. — " The new nurse in the North Gallery has voluntarily told me this morning that she dares not remain in the North Gallery any longer."

(Signed)   " E. P. CHARLESWORTH."

If, then, the staff of attendants was insufficient, how could I be blamed, or remonstrated with by the physician, who himself acknowledges this inefficiency in such direct terms ?

But why am I thus attacked ? Why am I thus unjustly injured, having given no offence ? The subjoined extract*

* " But my especial object in writing to you at present, is thus publicly to thank Dr Charlesworth, for his honourable avowal, at the late dinner of the Provincial Medical and Surgical Association at Hull, of the justness of my claims ; and also, Dr John Conolly, for his kind and handsome mention of my services. It cannot fail to be gratifying to myself to have their public testimony to the fact,

(see note) from my letter to the *Lancet* of September 6th, 1850, will prove that I had no hostility or " professional jealousy," as Mr Pierce terms it, with respect to Dr Charlesworth ;—on the contrary, that I nourished every good and grateful feeling towards him. But when a man turns round, contradicts his own previous testimony, and insinuates what he cannot prove, and dares not openly avow, as Dr Charlesworth does in his two last letters to the *Lancet,* to what gratitude* does this line of conduct entitle him?

After this explanation, I shall treat all attacks from the same quarter with the contempt they deserve. My opponents, however bitter their present enmity, cannot erase from the journals of the Lincoln Asylum the indelible testimonies therein given by themselves to the facts that I " broached the original and invaluable idea" of total abolition; that I first demonstrated its practicability; that I " *effected results* honourable to myself and beyond the hopes of the Board;" and that, as Dr Charlesworth truly states in his entry of October, 1841, I " *succeeded in my object.*"

I conclude with a letter from Dr John Forbes, containing his testimony, and that of Dr Conolly on the matter :—

" 12 Old Burlington street, Jan. 6, 1851.

" Sir,—Please put my name down as a subscriber of one guinea to Mr Hill's testimonial. In advocating the claims of Dr Conolly, I have never over-looked those of Mr Hill as the originator of the non-restraint system in our

---

that I originated the system which Dr Conolly and others have since carried out upon so large a scale, and with such beneficial results—results which will ensure the permanent continuance of the system of non-restraint, when the author shall be forgotten in the chambers of the grave."

* It is singular that Mr Pierce, when accusing me of ingratitude to Dr Charlesworth, should have quoted a paragraph from the Preface to my Lecture, and actually suppressed the succeeding sentence in which I acknowledged his assistance :—" To his" (Dr Charlesworth's) steady support under many difficulties, I owe chiefly the success which has attended *my plans and labours.*" This suppression is not less singular than dishonest.

Asylums. In proof that Dr Conolly himself does justice to Mr Hill's merits, Dr Conolly suggested to me, long ago, whether some portion of *his* subscription might not appropriately be devoted to the recognition of Mr Hill's claims. This, of course, could not be done.

" Yours faithfully,

" JOHN FORBES."

" Rev. J. Daniel."

I have the honour to be

My Lords, Ladies, and Gentlemen,

Your faithful servant,

ROBERT GARDINER HILL.

Eastgate-House,
Lincoln, May 23, 1851.

(Appendix E.)

Another extraordinary and inconsistent attack, by
the Editor of the ' Lancet,' in direct opposition to all his previous testimony.—Speeches
of Richard Sutton Harvey Esq., and Richard
Mason, Esq., Governors of the Lincoln
Lunatic Asylum, upon the sudden and
violent opposition of the ' Lancet ' of Nov.
5th, 1853.—Refusal of the Editor of the
' Lancet ' to insert the author's replies.—
Opinions of the ' Stamford Mercury ' (local
county paper), and of the Editor of the
' Medical Circular ';—Letters of Drs Wingett
and H. van Leeuwen.

1853, *November 5.*—' *Lancet*,' Leading Article. — " The
longing for posthumous fame is one of the purest and
noblest incentives which can stimulate an honourable
ambition. This desire to prolong our earthly existence, and
to live in the memories of our fellow-men is akin to that
holier aspiration which carries the soul into the realms of
immortality. The man who is animated by this passion will
surely spurn whatever is unworthy ; he will strive to link
his name with the remembrance of good deeds, and of
benefits conferred upon humanity. Mankind should hold
such men in honour. Posterity, as it is the inheritor of the
fruit of their labours, should regard itself as the special
guardian of their fame. Ingratitude and folly, baseness and

dishonesty, are the terms which would fitly represent the conduct of those, who by overt assent, or by no less culpable silence, should connive at defrauding the great and good men who have departed from amongst us of the honour they had righteously achieved. It were base cowardice on the part of posterity to consent to so foul a theft. As for the despoiler who would rob the illustrious dead of the credit of their discoveries, and of their title to the lasting gratitude of mankind, he must be held to be guilty of a great crime, and the author of the most flagitious treason against society!

" Since the ever-memorable revolution in our prison-discipline, brought about through the labours of Howard, the Philanthropist, no event has marked more honourably, or more unmistakeably, the progress of social amelioration in recent times than the remarkable transition from brutality to benevolence in the treatment of lunatics, initiated, in 1792, by the enlightened courage of Pinel. The day when this great apostle of humanity struck off the chains which had up to that time bound the bodies and crushed the afflicted minds of the insane, forms an era in the annals of science, and is one of the proudest records of which our profession can boast. That day is marked by the most emphatic and striking recognition of the rights of humanity; and it has ever since been blessed by successive achievements in the same cause, only less useful and less meritorious because they are but the fruit and the development of the rich and prolific germ planted by Pinel.

" Those labourers in the field of humanity and science who have followed in the track laid down by Pinel, will share in the honour rendered to him. Posterity will not fail to award to them that measure of applause which is justly due to those who ably and zealously endeavour to fulfil a noble mission.

" Pinel bequeathed to his successors the task of extending and perfecting that revolution in which he took the first and

S

most important step. His was the parent idea. Let no man lay a sacrilegious hand upon his grave ; let no man seek to pluck a single leaf from the wreath of honour which surrounds his glorious name,—a name revered by science, endeared to humanity, and blessed by the suffering.

" But the most appropriate tribute that we can bring to his memory and his worth, is to associate with his name the names of those who have struggled, with patient courage and enlightened zeal, against the active opposition of party malevolence and the passive weight of ignorance, to build up the edifice, of which the plan and the foundations were broadly laid by the master-architect. In our endeavours to estimate truly the relative claims of those who have taken part in this work, the foremost merit must be accorded to priority. Far deeper is the stamp of originality in his mind, far greater is his courage, who recognises the value of a great truth at a time when it is all but universally despised, than the originality and the courage of him who catches the bright thought at the turn of the tide, and swims down with the current of opinion. The nearer we ascend to the time of Pinel, the closer we come into conflict with the arrayed opposition of benighted ignorance, of inveterate custom,—and there is no custom so inveterate or so obstinate as that of cruelty,—and of deaf indifference. He who is firm in faith, and resolute in purpose, at such a time, although he may leave but few visible physical marks of his service behind him, is entitled to far greater praise than is he who comes later into the field, and, when slow conviction has wrought upon the minds of men, carries into final execution the reforms pointed out and prepared by his predecessors.

" If we search the history of the mode in which lunatics have been treated in this country with scrupulous impartiality, and a conscientious regard to the principles we have expressed, we shall find no individual who has earned for himself an equal claim to the respect of his fellow-citizens, or who has achieved so good a title to take rank next to Pinel himself, as the late Dr Charlesworth, who recently died, after having held for more than thirty years the post of Visiting-Physician to the Lincoln Asylum.

"At the time when this most estimable man and accomplished physician entered upon his career, scarcely an advance had been made to establish in England that system of moral treatment which Pinel had sought to substitute for the most brutal physical coercion. Early, indeed, and because early, doubly honourable, were the exertions of Dr Tuke, of the York Retreat: useful and fruitful was the lesson he taught by example of the safety and success of treating the insane with humanity. But then, and we are reluctant to qualify our praise of one who must ever hold a foremost place in the esteem of mankind, the difficulties which Dr Tuke had to encounter were of a different and far less arduous kind than those which for long years encumbered the path of Dr Charlesworth. In the York Retreat Dr Tuke was absolute. He was the uncontrolled master to carry his benevolent designs into effect. Not so Dr Charlesworth. He had first of all to uplift the dead weight of error, of prejudice, and of fear; to make proselytes to a doctrine which was then new, and which to many who heard it sounded like heresy; which to many more appeared like the dream of an enthusiastic visionary. Dr Charlesworth's first labour was to impart his views to a large body of independent gentlemen, impressed with a serious sense of the deep responsibility which rested upon them, as the official governors of the Lincoln Asylum, should mischance or failure attend upon any change of system they might sanction. It is not the least significant tribute to the character of Dr Charlesworth, or the least convincing proof of his great qualities and earnestness of purpose, that he succeeded so completely in this task, and that he was able to mould so many of the leading gentlemen of the county of Lincoln into willing assistants and partners in his plan. It is not too much to say that, from the year 1819 down to the time of his death, almost every successive improvement in the construction and management of the Lincoln Asylum had originated with Dr Charlesworth, and been carried out under his immediate inspiration. In 1819, at Lincoln, and for many long years after in other public asylums, and still we greatly fear in some, it was the practice to permit the attendants or keepers, as they were then appropriately called, to fetter and chain up the patients at their discretion. The first record of the active zeal of Dr Charlesworth is contained in an order of the Board commanding—' That the attendants and servants never presume to use any degree of restraint or violence without the consent of the director.'

" By this regulation the treatment of the patients was at once brought within the sole control of the medical officers. From this time forward we trace, from year to year, and almost from day to day, the most gratifying proofs of the gradual unfolding of Dr Charlesworth's great design. The fulfilment of that design involved the necessity of a total subversion of the constitution of the Asylum, an entire change in the construction of the building, and the introduction of a totally different system of classifying and treating the patients. The building that was adapted for a prison or a menagerie, the sole contrivance in which was directed to secure the unhappy inmates by the various appliances of physical restraint, was necessarily a place ill adapted for the action of the opposite system. The abolition of physical restraint implies, as a logical consequence, the substitution of moral control. During the slow disappearance of the physical ' impedimeta,' and the equally slow and painful task of eradicating the brutal notions of the keepers, and of training them to new modes of thought, we can only look for gradual and successive steps in the progress of amelioration.

"Dr Charlesworth early felt that his plan must prove abortive, if he could not change the entire structure and machinery of the Asylum. The grounds of the Asylum were deficient of means to prevent the escape of the patients. But then the patients were all locked up or secured by fetters! What need of walls? Dr Charlesworth's next object, therefore, was 'to encircle the front garden with a low wall, with a deep-sunk fence within.' This preliminary arrangement completed, physical freedom and exercise became possible.

"In 1821 another great advance was made. Up to that time the epileptic, the melancholic, the idiotic, the incurable, and the convalescent all associated together. The construction of the building was again the obstacle to improvement. Dr Charlesworth pointed out this difficulty in his reports. 'I am aware that the necessary improvements cannot be effected in the present exhausted state of the finances. On them, however, the character and support of the institution must eventually rest, as involving the security, the health, and the restoration of the patients.' 'Some of the men,' he urged, 'are kept almost constantly in manacles, or apart in the maniacal cells, to protect the weak and quiet from the outrages of the strong.' In April, 1827, Dr Charlesworth had matured a plan for altering the buildings, so as to admit of classification, and a committee was appointed, of which he was a member, and whose first step was to adopt his plan.

"The strongest proof to our minds of the large and enlightened views of Dr Charlesworth is found in his eagerness to court public inspection. There is no index so sure of abuse as mystery; there is no corrective influence so wholesome as publicity. 'My jealousy on the point of facility of inspection is extreme. Viewing this privilege as one of the principal safeguards of the patients, I regard every step towards its diminution as a step towards mal-treatment, and every impediment thrown in its way as introductory to abuse.' This was written in 1828. How far in advance of the authorities of metropolitan Bethlehem, who, down to 1852, shrank, as well they might, from the public gaze! The consequence of Dr Charlesworth's letter was a series of resolutions of the Board, calculated to ensure every facility for inspection. They also ordered 'that every instrument of restraint, *when not in use*, be hung up in a place distinctly appropriated (to that purpose), so that the number and nature of such instruments in use at any time may appear.' In 1829, we find the following passage in the minutes, well illustrating the tendency of the reformatory measures in progress, and clearly expressing the consummation in perspective : ' The governors have particularly directed their views to the subject of coercion and restraints, well aware of their injurious consequences to the patients.' Various steps towards the diminution and restriction of restraints are then reported. Handcuffs and strait-waistcoats of the more objectionable description were destroyed. The house-surgeon had long been ordered to keep a journal for entering the particulars of every case in which he resorted to coercion. In 1831, the Board pointedly made the following declaration—namely, 'that the fair measure of a superintendent's ability in the treatment of the insane will be found in the small number of restraints which are imposed.' In 1832 we find that Dr Charlesworth reported that 'a patient had been kept under continual restraint on account of the insecurity of the inner male court. This inconvenience has been met by a slight alteration of the windows of the adjoining gallery, which had afforded a passage to the roof. . . . An order has been made to procure ' strong dresses ' for patients disposed to tear their clothes,' thus superseding the ' belt ' and ' muff.' A substitute for that ingenious instrument of torture, the ' hobbles,' was also suggested by the physician.

" In April, 1833, the Board 'has pleasure in being able to state that the recent alterations in the buildings and courts are found to answer all the intentions of the governors.' On the same occasion, it is broadly stated, that ' it is *unceasingly an object in this Institution to dispense with or to improve as much as possible the instruments of restraint.*' The governing idea ever present in the mind of Dr Charlesworth is manifest. It was further exemplified in 1834 by another contrivance, which Dr Conolly afterwards adopted. Dr Charlesworth observed that, ' as the disposition of some patients to tear their blankets is occasionally a cause of their being confined by the wrists at night, he recommended that in such cases the blankets should be enclosed within strong Russia sheeting, quilted.' In the same year, and with the same view of guarding against the resort to restraint, a system of night-watching was arranged; and on the 21st of July a further destruction of instruments of restraint was ordered. In September, a further security was provided by placing glazed doors at the ends of the galleries, so as to admit of complete supervision of the patients and attendants by the house-surgeon.

" It would be tedious, however instructive, to recite all the various suggestions and improvements conceived and executed under the guidance of Dr Charlesworth, all tending to the attainment of his great end, down to this period. In 1835, his arrangements were rapidly approaching to perfection; the manifest physical obstructions had almost disappeared; the realization of his long-cherished and long-pursued idea, through a tried course of experience, of observation, and of contrivance, now become practicable, was at hand. He had triumphed over the stubbornness of ignorance, the hesitation of fear, the meanness of parsimony, the jealousy of colleagues, and the resistance of sloth. Successive house-surgeons had caught his enthusiasm, and nobly seconded his policy. The career of each was marked by progressive success in diminishing restraint in exact proportion to the advancing improvements in the buildings and subsidiary arrangements. Let us pass in rapid review the chief reforms and the gradual evanescence of restraint.

" The complete means of classification afforded by the improved construction of the building.

" The dormitory under night-watch.

" The increase in the number of well-selected attendants.

" The supervision by means of sashed doors.

" The wholesome influence of public inspection.

" The open depository for the instruments of restraint.

" The official authority required for each instance of their application, and the subsequent registry.

" The use of strong dresses.

" The abundant exercise in the open air.

" The total abstinence from fermented liquors.

" All these improvements had been effected, and all these arrangements were in operation. In 1832, Dr Charlesworth was enabled to report that ' the Register of Restraints shows a continual diminution in their number.' On the 10th of August, 1834, the house-visitor reported that ' not a single male patient had been under restraint since the 16th of July, and not one female patient since the 1st of August, and then only for a few hours ;' and in 1835, the Board took the opportunity of specially recording their sense of the merit of Mr Hadwen, the house-surgeon, by expressing ' their high approbation of the very small proportion of instances of restraint which had occurred under his care.'

" But then, in July, 1835, there enters upon the scene a man of such lofty pretensions that, were the world to estimate them by the standard he has set up, certainly not only Dr Charlesworth, but Conolly, and Pinel himself, must hide their diminished heads. To Mr Hadwen there succeeds Mr Gardiner Hill, now Mayor of Lincoln, and proprietor of a private asylum. Let us at once broadly state the claim of Mr Hill; or, perhaps we should fail to do justice to the modesty which is not the least conspicuous ornament of his merit, if we did not allow Mr Hill to state that claim in his own unassuming language. Mr Hill made a speech, which a journal took the pains to report. There occurred this sentence : ' He (Mr Hill) was bound to acknowledge that the system (of non-restraint) did, *to some extent*, (!) originate with himself.' There was modesty, but it was not Mr Hill's. This gentleman indignantly repudiates qualified praise. Pinel, Conolly, Tuke, Charlesworth, are not worthy to tie his shoe-strings. Mr Hill must be the ' bright particular star,' eclipsing every orb of lesser magnitude in the effulgence of his rays. Mr Hill thus accosts the unfaithful editor : ' Now, the words "to some extent " were never uttered by me, and seem to throw a doubt upon my being, as the records of the Lincoln Asylum indisputably and indelibly prove me to be, the *sole author and originator* of the total abolition or non-restraint system in the treatment of lunatics.' This merit is ' one which no one else can claim, and of which I shall not allow any one to rob me.' Mr Hill is as sensitive as he is modest. He shall not be robbed ; but the world and the profession will not be so ungrateful as to forget that the memory of the dead has also rights that must not be despoiled.

" But what are these ' indisputable and indelible records' to which Mr Hill appeals ? Not surely those which relate the history of the Asylum and its rise under the fostering genius of Dr Charlesworth for many long years prior to the era of Mr Hill in 1835! No. These are of trifling moment. Nothing had been done ; none of those necessary antecedents of the system which we have quoted are entitled to the smallest merit. The whole system, the whole plan, burst forth from the brain of Mr Hill *totus teres atque rotundus;* no preparation from others—no room for future improvements. A Minerva from the labouring skull of Jove! Such is the announcement of this world-famous discovery. It is contained in a report dated April 12, 1837:—' The present house-surgeon has expressed his own belief, founded on experience in this house, that it may be possible to conduct an institution for the insane without having recourse to the employment of any instrument of restraint whatsoever.' Hear this—but forget that Pinel and Charlesworth had lived before the advent of Mr Hill! Mr Hill's origination then consists in ' expressing a belief.' What if this belief were premature ? What if it were but the frothy conceit of a rash, short-sighted man ? What if it were nullified, discredited, and belied by the subsequent ' experience' of the very man who gave it utterance! In 1837, Mr Hill entertained a ' belief,' which he has subsequently elevated to the dignity of a ' discovery.' In April, 1840, within three short years of his ' discovery,' there occurs this self-convicting record in his journal :—

" ' Nurse Corston came to my room . . . . and told me that she could not remain in the gallery if C. A— was allowed to get up, as, in the event of an outbreak, the other nurses would not dare to give assistance.'

" Where is Mr Hill's faith ? where his ' discovery?'

" ' *I directed Corston to place C. A—— under restraint.* On entering the gallery . . . . I found this patient quietly putting on her clothes, and she appeared orderly . . . . Everything being ready, the patient was held by two nurses. The *belt* was then put on loosely. The moment I attempted to secure the wrists a struggle commenced, the *wrist-locks* being seized by the patient and locked at each attempt I made . . . . At length she was thrown down and overpowered'!

" Behold the ' discovery!' Admire the ' originator' of non-restraint ! Let no one ' rob him ' of his title !

" Shall we say more ? Yes ! Justice as to the rare nobility

of mind of Dr Charlesworth requires us to proceed. Dr Charlesworth was never sparing in his praise of others. He had found that the cause he had ever at heart was progressing. He grudged to no one, however subordinate his services, a lavish share in his own merit. In 1838, *before* the above deplorable instance of Mr Hill's failure, Dr Charlesworth had stated in an official report,—

" ' The bold conception of pushing the mitigation of restraint to the extent of actually and formally abolishing the practice, mentioned in the last Report as due to Mr Hill, the house-surgeon, seems to be justified by the following abstract, &c.'

" This is another ' indelible record' to which Mr Hill appeals. He seeks to dispute with Dr Charlesworth the honour of *originating* the system of non-restraint. What a rare stroke of strategy if he can cite the testimony of Dr Charlesworth in support of his own pretension against Dr Charlesworth! Fortunately even Dr Charlesworth could not thus divest himself of his title to renown, nor make an ' originator' out of Mr Hill. But Mr Hill relies upon this testimony. We therefore entreat every candid mind to weigh well its import, and to decide whether the words, ' a bold conception, mentioned as due to Mr Hill, and which *seems* to be justified,' afford ' indisputable' evidence of Mr Hill's *originality*, or whether these words, and Mr Hill's construction of them do but prove the generosity of Dr Charlesworth, and that that generosity has been abused.

" But, if Dr Charlesworth could indeed renounce his own claim, what is still the testimony of those entitled to credit? To whom does Dr Conolly award the praise of having led the way in that path which he has himself so honourably trodden? We extract the following from a letter to Dr Charlesworth :—

" ' For I never forget that it is to *you* that I and all of us are indebted for being roused to useful and benevolent exertion in behalf of the insane.'

" And this will be the testimony of every one who shall honestly trace the history of the subject. Shall it be that Dr Charlesworth broke up the virgin and ungrateful soil, that he tilled the land, sowed the wheat, rooted out the weeds, and nurtured the plant, through every adversity, to ripeness, and that a subordinate, employed at a late period of the work, shall reap the full harvest of honour and applause?

" But a testimonial has been got up to Mr Hill. Does that testimonial bear witness to the justice of Mr Hill's claim? The world will interpret it otherwise. It records the good-natured weakness of many; the personal feelings of some ; the ignorance of others: it leaves Mr Hill's pretensions to be settled by the sterner and more impartial criticism of truth.

" We have felt it our duty to subject this matter to a careful scrutiny. Hesitation upon such an occasion would be to sanction injustice towards one who has gone from amongst us. To be negligent in this duty would be an abdication of the greatest privilege of the press—to defend the memory of those who can no longer defend themselves, and to hold out to the admiration and imitation of mankind the noble example of great difficulties manfully overcome.

" In the Lincoln Asylum, the scene of Dr Charlesworth's philanthropic struggle and success, it is proposed to erect a bust in commemoration of his services. It would not be fitting that this memorial should be raised by local subscriptions alone. Dr Charlesworth's services were not local, but of national and of cosmopolitan importance: they should have a commensurate recognition."

1853, *November* 9.—From the *Stamford Mercury and Lincolnshire Times.*—" Lincoln Municipality.—Mr Harvey reminded the Council that on Mr Hill's elevation to office, he spoke of him as being well known to science and humanity, as the originator of the non-restraint system in lunacy. He would not have alluded to that subject, but for the attack so recently made upon the Mayor of Lincoln, at the eleventh hour of his retiring from office, in the pages of the *Lancet*. He felt surprised and great regret that those pages, in which Mr Hill had so repeatedly and successfully defeated his opponents, had again opened the question. He felt certain that the high-minded editor of that journal would afford Mr Hill a fair opportunity to meet his antagonists. Mr Harvey (turning towards Mr Hill) continued. I would recommend you, Mr Hill, to bear up as nobly under your present trying circumstances as you have always done. The sophistry of your opponents, the hatred of those who were your early friends, and who are now your bitterest enemies —who seem to have laid themselves at your heels, and are determined to hound you to the death—shall die out with them. When they shall be laid in their graves, and you, Mr Hill, shall be resting quietly and honourably in your grave, the evidence you will leave behind you of your reputation, is sure and certain. And wherever non-restraint in lunacy shall be known or spoken of, it shall ever be associated with your name and the city of Lincoln, and you shall take rank amongst the noblest philanthropists. (Cheers.) Mr Hill said it was gratifying to him to find that his official services during the past year had given satisfaction. * * * * Mr Harvey's remarks he thought exceedingly opportune, especially as his (Mr Hill's) claims to the honour of being the originator of the system of non-restraint had been so recently impugned. He had defended those claims at considerable cost to himself, but, he believed, to the satisfaction of the public. He was, however, again the subject of a gross and calumnious attack, which had appeared in the *Lancet*, for the purpose of enabling his

late opponents to erect a statue to the memory of the late
Dr Charlesworth, as the originator of his (Mr R. G. Hill's)
system. He felt confident his friends and fellow-citizens
would never allow such an act of injustice to pass without
remonstrance. He had in his possession indisputable proof
that he originated the system, and that he was innocent of
the charges made against him. He defended his claims
during the life-time of Dr Charlesworth, who declared, at
a large meeting of the Medical and Surgical Association,
held at Hull, that the 'real honour belonged to Mr Hill of
the Lincoln Asylum.'

" The Town Clerk (Richard Mason, Esq., a Governor
of the Lincoln Lunatic Asylum for twenty-three years)
alluded to the attack made upon Mr Hill in the pages of
the *Lancet*. It was to be deplored that such an article
should appear at the present season, although it showed how
embittered the writer was against Mr Hill. He (the Town
Clerk) did not think much of the article itself,—it was
empty, inflated, and displayed great hostility to Mr Hill.
It was full of sound and fury, which meant nothing. It
was a thesis on the dishonour of robbing the dead. The
question was, did the honour of originating the system of non-
restraint belong to the dead? Did the late Dr Charlesworth
ever question Mr Hill's claim? Why, he delivered a lecture
at the Mechanics' Institution in this city, in the life-time
of Dr Charlesworth, in which he (Mr. Hill) spoke of
himself *as being the originator of the system*, and this lecture
was submitted to Dr Charlesworth before it was delivered.
Those parts relating to Mr Hill, as being the originator
of non-restraint, were untouched by the late Doctor himself.
At a meeting of the Medical Provincial Association, held
at Hull, subsequently, when Dr Conolly, Dr Charlesworth,
and others interested, were present, on Mr Hill's health
being proposed, Dr Charlesworth disclaimed the merit of
being the originator of the system of total non-restraint,

and gave the credit to Mr Hill. Recent proceedings were more like the friends of the dead endeavouring to rob the living of the honour to which they were justly entitled. The extracts in the article, from the Asylum minutes, contained nothing which negatived Mr Hill's claims. The question was *whether Mr Hill did not come forward first to do away with restraint altogether?* Prior to Mr Hill, Mr Hadwen had declared that it was absurd to suppose that they could do without mechanical restraint altogether. The article in the *Lancet* was the last kick which a philanthropic man could receive from envious persons. When time had passed on, Mr Hill would receive his reward, and be placed in a niche of fame, as one of those who had benefitted his country in the cause of humanity. (Cheers.)"

1853, *November* 11.—*Stamford Mercury.* — " The last number of the *Lancet* revives a question which the *Lancet* itself settled long since—the right of the origination of the entire abolition of instrumental restraint in the management of lunatics. The article in question would entitle the author to the presidential chair of a Jesuits' College. It is a masterpiece of sophistry. It leaps over all evidence—all documentary testimony. The Asylum records prove that the late Dr Charlesworth zealously laboured to mitigate the horrors of instrumental restraint, but that the total and unconditional abolition of restraint was never entertained by Dr Charlesworth, or any of the Lincoln Asylum management, until it was broached by Mr Hill, and its practicability demonstrated by him."

1853, *November* 5.—*Medical Circular*, Leading Article. —" Two months ago a certain gentleman sent to us for publication a series of printed documents, containing a letter and appendices, which had been put into circulation more than two years prior to our being favoured with the communication, and which, had they been accepted, would have occupied together about a dozen columns of the *Medical Circular;* and a letter accompanying these documents, offering to PAY us for the accorded privilege of publication. On perusing the papers we discovered that they disclosed an elaborate attempt to asperse and degrade the character of Mr Robert Gardiner Hill, Mayor of Lincoln : we, therefore, disdained to accept the paltry bribe, and resolved that our pages should never be made the medium of purchased vituperation. Our advertising sheet is the proper place for a marketable transaction.

" We were not, however, surprised to observe, in the last number of the *Lancet,* that the documents we rejected had been received and embodied in a leading article by the Editor of that highminded and scrupulous periodical. We know well that this paper has been, for a long time, the receptacle for the literary offal shunted aside by ourselves and other organs of the medical press, and we could not therefore feel astonished that the overtures we repelled the *Lancet* had eagerly embraced. We should like to know how much has been paid into its treasury in requital of the slavish service it has rendered to the miserable faction whose cause it espouses.

" The occasion of aiding in the object of founding a memorial to that virtuous and amiable man, Dr Charlesworth, was little suited for heaping slander upon the professional name of Mr Hill. Were Dr Charlesworth alive he would have indignantly rebuked the writer who could so wantonly desecrate his revered name as to pervert the hour of his honour to the base purposes of party faction, and to make it the signal for pouring out the vials of envy, hatred, and all uncharitableness on the head of a former colleague and friend. We think the Editor, if he have any shame, must, by this time, be thoroughly disgusted with his work."

From the *Medical Circular*, November 23, 1853.—Leading Article :—

" THE NON-RESTRAINT SYSTEM IN THE TREATMENT OF LUNACY.

" Invariable experience attests that no great discovery in science, nor any important improvement in the methods or appliances of art, has been made in entire independence of the meditations and labours of other men. The most penetrating genius has not been able to see far in advance of others experimenting in the same field ; and most commonly the loftiest scientific achievement has been either a sagacious generalisation of the labours of the predecessors, or the discovery of the last link wanting to complete the chain of facts connecting, in unbroken series, a variety of physical phenomena to their fundamental and regulating cause. The last proof, fortuitous or contrived, easy or laborious, enables the fortunate discoverer to complete a grand induction, suspected, foreshadowed, and, probably, believed by other men, but never before demonstrated ; hence he derives his title to all the honours which the world has been accustomed to award to successful genius. The announcer of a new law, clearly exhibited, becomes the recipient of the smaller fame of his predecessors. He absorbs their labours, and is reputed as the master of the vineyard, whose fruits have become his property by the superior ascendancy of his character, and by the general consent of the world.

" The fact that many minds are usually employed in the endeavour to attain the same result, and have generally aided, in a greater or less degree, in its accomplishment, has frequently led to the detraction of the fair fame of the man to whom the credit of the conclusion justly belongs. As soon as the wonder of the new announcement has subsided, numerous candidates for priority gradually assert their pretensions, or are, by envious and carping critics, disentombed from their unhonoured graves to dispute the possession of the bays with the rightful owner.

T

" Newton was not allowed to enjoy his fame in peace, and his quarrel with Liebnitz divided and convulsed the scientific world. Watt's claim to be the author of the steam-engine has been attributed to Newcomen, and, failing his pretensions, to the mad Marquis of Worcester ; yet Watt's name will be associated with the steam-engine to the end of time, because he concluded and perfected the labours of all his predecessors. They were no more than slaves carrying bricks and straw for the great master-builder. Attempts have been made to deprive Columbus of the credit of discovering the Western Continent, because some wandering Norsemen, and men greater than they—John and Sebastian Cabot—had discovered Greenland before him ; yet, while we allow the Cabots' claim to glory, we shall not seek to diminish by a single leaf the wreath of laurel with which the head of Columbus has been crowned by the concurrent applause of all nations.

" In our own profession the same cavillers have gnawed at the reputation of the illustrious Harvey, and professed to have detected, by their microscopic criticism, a prior claimant to the honour of discovering the circulation of the blood ; and, in our own day, the merit that belongs to Marshall Hall has been vehemently disputed, and his brilliant generalisations given to an obscurer name.

" We despise the miserable critics who, in the pursuit of their craft, are ever on the watch to despoil a man of his just honour ; and who seek to prevent an individual becoming great by dividing the credit due to him among a herd of small pretenders. These snarlers have at all times infected the republic of science, and yelped in concert at the heels of every individual who has done a good or a great thing, and has been fortunate enough to acquire the respect of his fellows ; they sicken at the sight of superior ability, and die of envy to think that any man but themselves should achieve a title to the lasting gratitude of mankind.

" This is the position in which we now find Mr Robert

Gardiner Hill placed in relation to his critics. Despite the most convincing evidence that he was the first person who thoroughly appreciated and proclaimed the truth and safety of the 'non-restraint' system in the treatment of lunacy, these malignant antagonists continue to carp at his pretensions, and endeavour to deter him from defending his honour by loading his name with base insinuations, odious charges, and despicable calumnies. We blushed for the honour of our common profession when we read the language in which the rancorous traducer of the *Lancet* discharged his venom on the name of Mr Gardiner Hill; yet more when the cowardly scribe deprived that gentleman of the opportunity of cleansing it of the pollution in the pages of the journal in which the perverted statements and malicious accusations had appeared.

" By what code of justice can the *Lancet* feel authorised to publish its calumnies against a private individual, and forbid him afterwards the opportunity of repelling the disingenuous and false charges in the presence of the same tribunal before which they were made? The refusal of the *Lancet* to publish the reply of Mr Gardiner Hill to its elaborate slanders, is one of the most dastardly acts that have ever disgraced our literature. Indignant at the treatment Mr Hill has received, we are resolved that he shall have a hearing, and we are convinced that it will redound to his great honour, and to the shame and confusion of his enemies.

" Let Mr Hill be assured that the good feeling and the sense of justice of every independent member of the profession are on his side, and will support him against his calumniators. That he is entitled to be considered as the *originator* of the system of ' non-restraint' is incontestable, as will appear on an honest examination of the evidence ; and although his claim is denied by the *Lancet,* our indignation is not directed so much against such opposition, as matter of opinion, as against the bad taste and malignancy with which the attack was begun, and the cowardice and injustice with which the defence was disallowed. Why did not the *Lancet* publish Mr Hill's reply ? Clearly because it contained a triumphant refutation of the Editor's dishonest allegations, and would have necessitated an apology for his detraction. Mr Hill is charged by implication in the *Lancet* with ' ingratitude and folly, baseness and dishonesty,' and yet this Editor, who is of course the reverse of all that, is ' ungrateful, foolish, base, and dishonest ' forbids Mr Hill's defence from appearing in his pages !

" It is quite possible that Dr Daquin, who preceded Pinel, and Pinel, who worked anterior to Dr Veitch, and Dr Veitch who anticipated Dr Tuke, and Dr Tuke, who set an example to Dr Charlesworth, and Dr Charlesworth himself may all alike, while doing their utmost to mitigate the use of instruments of restraint, have been sceptical of the practicability of the entire abolition of instrumental resources. Pinel himself, the far-seeing, the philanthropic, and the firm, would have regarded a philanthropist as insane who should have come to him and advised the entire disuse of coercive instruments in his Asylum. Even when Mr Robert Gardiner Hill announced the discovery, it was received with disbelief and encountered scoffs and contempt; but the perseverance and courage of Dr Conolly, demonstrated on an extensive scale, the practicability of Mr Hill's great principle; and now it is the wretched aim of the jeerers and calumniators to deprive Mr Hill of the honour a discovery so grand and startling, has naturally attracted.

" They will not succeed. The merit of introducing the system of non-restraint is as unquestionably ascribable to Mr Hill, as the honour of discovering the north west passage will belong to Captain M'Clure, should that gallant officer happily succeed in his enterprise. What though the possibility of making the passage has been believed for centuries,—that a Ross, a Parry, a Beechy, a Back, a Franklin, and many more brave officers, have expended their energies and wasted their lives in the attempt; that the most practicable routes have been delineated in the charts, and the difficulties of the adventure have been gradually reduced, still the fact remains to be proved; and should Captain M'Clure be the fortunate man to solve the problem of ages, he will have satisfied the ardent expectations of his countrymen, whose admiration and gratitude will acknowledge him as the discoverer of the passage, and a long posterity will do honour to his sagacity, his intrepidity, and his perseverance. Yet Mr Hill's claim to honour is even stronger than that of Captain M'Clure; for he discovered what does not appear to have been surmised by any of his predecessors : viz., the practicability of an entire abolition of instruments of restraint;—and he proved his proposition.

" There are only two persons whose claims can be set up in opposition to those of Mr Hill; those persons are the predecessor of Mr Hill in the Asylum—Mr Hadwen; and the visiting physician, the late Dr Charlesworth. What says Mr Hadwen on the subject ? In a letter addressed to the Editor of the *Lancet* in 1841, he remarks—

" ' Restraint forms the very basis and principle on which the sound treatment of lunatics is founded. The judicious and appropriate adaptation of the various modifications of this powerful means to the peculiarities of each case of insanity, comprises a large portion of the curative regimen of the scientific and rational practitioner; in his hands it is a remedial agent of the very first importance ; and it appears to me that it is about as likely to be dispensed with in the case of mental diseases, as that the various articles of the materia medica will be altogether dispensed with in the case of the bodily.'—(Mr Hadwen's letter to the *Times*, Jan. 25th, 1841.)

" Here we are favoured with an express declaration in

favour of the ' *principle* ' of ' *restraint ;* ' and in another place
Mr Hadwen charges Mr Gardiner Hill with ' rashness ' for
avowing the 'principle' of ' non-restraint.' So much for
the claims of Mr Hadwen !

"What says Dr Charlesworth ? In the course of his
speech at the dinner of the Provincial Medical and Surgical
Association, held at Hull, August 16th, 1850, he attested
the right of Mr Hill in these words:—' The *real honour* of
FIRST INTRODUCING the SYSTEM is due to Mr Hill ! '

"Again, what say the Governors of the Asylum ? In
the Memorandum Book we find this paragraph, bearing date
Oct. 9, 1849 : ' The entire absence of restraint still continues, *to the high honour of the house-surgeon.*'

' EDW. FF. BROMHEAD.

' W. M. PIERCE.

' E. P. CHARLESWORTH.'

"And again, in the Report of Lincoln Asylum, 1849, this
sentence occurs with reference to the use of instruments of
restraint: 'At last, under these circumstances, the *idea occurred
to Mr Hill that no case of the kind whatsoever need exist;* and
in the practice he was determinedly supported by the Boards,
through every species of *opposition, exaggeration,* and *misrepresentation,* WITHIN the institution and WITHOUT.'

"After this, let the paltry scribblers of the *Lancet* write
on if they dare. Mr Hill's reputation stands upon an im-
moveable foundation, and will survive alike the low stra-
tagems of secret malice, and the more impudent attacks of
an unscrupulous and unjust press."

From the *Medical Circular*, November 23, 1853 :—

"MR ROBERT GARDINER HILL AND THE ' LANCET.'"

TO THE EDITOR OF THE ' MEDICAL CIRCULAR.'

"Sir,—My position as the originator of non-restraint
having been impugned in a violent and abusive article in

the *Lancet* of the 5th of November, I trust you will not refuse me the insertion of the following reply, which has also been forwarded to the *Lancet.*

"I have the honour to be, Sir,
"Your very faithful and obedient servant,
"ROBERT GARDINER HILL.
"Eastgate House, Lincoln, Nov. 14, 1853."

TO THE EDITOR OF THE 'LANCET.'

"Sir,—The acrimonious attack made upon me in the columns of your journal of the 5th inst. has surprised me much. The bitter personal feeling which characterises that attack might well excuse me from the trouble of a reply, especially as your readers can easily refer to the former pages of the *Lancet*, in which the justice of my claims has been repeatedly and fully vindicated. Upon calmer reflection, however, I consider it due to those gentlemen who subscribed to my testimonial, and to the public generally, to place before them the evidence of Dr Charlesworth and others connected with the Lincoln Asylum, upon the abolition of restraint in that institution. You say that 'Dr Charlesworth's first labour was to impart his views to a large body of independent gentlemen, impressed with a serious sense of the deep responsibility which rested upon them, as the Official Governors of the Lincoln Asylum, should mischance or failure attend upon any change of system they might sanction,' and you date this in 1819. What Dr Charlesworth's views were upon the subject of restraint in 1829, ten years after, may be gathered from the only publication* he ever wrote on the subject, in which he says (page 15), 'The modes of coercion are those which excite the least uneasiness, and have been most frequently a leathern belt, or a chain round the waist, with iron manacles for the wrists, attached to the belt or chain by a small chain

* *Remarks on the Treatment of the Insane*, by E. P. Charlesworth, M.D. 1829.

a few inches long. For patients who tear their clothes the "muff" is generally employed. Perhaps leather used in the dress of these patients might occasionally supersede the necessity of restraint. Some cases require the use of the strait-waistcoat; or, to prevent violent kicking, a restraint for the legs, called "hobbles," which allow the action of walking; but these and the strait-waistcoat are comparatively little employed. The average number of patients under personal restraint may be stated at from one to three in forty; sometimes not one for several weeks together.'
'The restraints employed have been almost entirely at the discretion of the director, always under his superintendence, and under the eyes of the physician and weekly visitor, whose attendance is frequent and casual. The use of distinct apartments prevent the necessity of placing patients under confinement during the night, except such as may be expected to injure themselves. Sometimes there are two or three; often not one for several months in succession. It would be an improvement that some public and accessible room should be set apart, in which should be hung up every instrument of restraint, without exception, labelled with separate numbers from No. 1 upwards, to correspond with similar labels and numbers on the walls, so as instantly to show how many of such instruments are in use at any time. Such an exposure would tend to diminish both the number and use of such instruments; would occasion them to be kept always clean, and not in the foul, hard, and unsupple state so uneasy to the patient; would cause the instruments to be of the slightest and least harsh form that could be safely used; and by calling the attention of visitors to their shape and object, would no doubt lead to improvements.'

"In 1830, the year following the publication of this work, 27,113 hours were passed under restraint by patients in the Lincoln Asylum.

"In 1842 I was attacked by several anonymous correspondents in the *Lancet*, and by Dr Finch, of Laverstock House. The following replies, written in the presence of Dr Charlesworth, and with his own autograph additions, proved that he never claimed to be the originator of a system which he knew and always avowed to belong to myself:—

TO THE EDITOR OF THE 'LANCET.'*

" ' Sir, — If your correspondents 'Exetasticos' and 'Quæstor' will favour myself and the public with their real names, I will be happy to reply to their communications through your journal. The acrimonious attacks to which my prominent position, as the originator of the total abolition of instrumental restraint in lunacy, have exposed me from its opponents, make it necessary that I should resort to this measure of *self*-protection from irresponsible antagonists.

" ' I am, Sir,
" ' Your obedient and faithful servant,
" ' ROBT. GARDINER HILL.

" ' Lincoln, July 23, 1842.' "

" ' Sir,—In the number of your journal, to which in your last you have referred me, I find a communication from Dr Finch, claiming as his own, not a total abolition of instrumental restraint in his establishment at Laverstock House, but a per centage of exemption from such means of coercing his patients. I ground the claim which I have made to the total abolition of instrumental restraint upon the fact of its having been abolished in the Lincoln Asylum, under my superintendence, in January, 1837.

---

* The words underlined in these letters are in Dr Charlesworth's own handwriting.

" ' It is true that in one single case since the above date, *viz.*, *in April*, 1840, a patient was instrumentally restrained *for eighteen hours*, through circumstances solely imputable to a disorganised state of the staff of attendants, and not to any failure in the system, *when* carried out in the manner laid down in my lecture, delivered June 21, 1838, and published in April, 1839. I still wait for a preclaimant to the system of totally abolishing instrumental restraint in the management of the insane.

" 'And now, Mr Editor, allow me to congratulate yourself and the public, and *especially* the insane, upon the happy turn which the debate upon this subject, occupying so many of your pages, has at length taken. Instead of hearing any longer of the impracticability, the futility, or the absurdity of the system, denominated by its opponents as 'utopian,' 'speculative,' 'peculative,' &c., &c., you have now in the field combatants for the honour of the invention.'

" The signature of Dr Charlesworth to the report of 1838 should seem to be sufficient to settle the question; but I have abundant evidence even without this. In a letter testimonial to myself, dated Nov. 26, 1838, Dr Charlesworth says—'He' (Mr Hill) 'has diligently applied all the means of amelioration placed at his disposal, and in so doing has *conceived and effected results* honourable to himself, and *beyond the hopes of the Board. The practice of restraint and coercion has disappeared under his management.*'

" Again, 1841, Jan. 23, there occurs the following entry by Dr Charlesworth in the 'Physician's Journal' of the Lincoln Asylum : 'The bold position taken by Mr Hill in his publication on the non-restraint system, assuming the practicability of a total abolition of instrumental restraint was not less sensible than sound. The present house-surgeon has taken a similar position as regards the abolition of solitary confinement, and I trust he will succeed in his object, *as Mr Hill has done in his own.'*

(Signed)   "E. P. CHARLESWORTH."

"Here Dr Charlesworth bears witness to the soundness of my views, and to my success in carrying them out. ' What a rare stroke of strategy, if he (Mr Hill) can cite the testimony of Dr Charlesworth in support of his own pretension, against Dr Charlesworth! fortunately, when, Dr Charlesworth could not thus divest himself of his title to renown, nor make an ' originator ' out of Mr Hill!' So runs the late attack upon me in the *Lancet;* let us hear, however, what Dr Charlesworth does actually make of me. If we refer to Dr Granville's ' Spas of England,' Midland Division, page 87, there occurs the following passages :—

" ' In speaking of a full and true execution of the plan of not coercing patients, applied to a large lunatic asylum in all cases of mental disturbance, no matter of what nature and degree, one is bound to defer the palm of originality and perseverance to Mr Hill, whose work on the subject has probably led the way to a totally new era in the management of insane persons.' * * * ' After a first introduction to the senior physician (Dr Charlesworth) of the (Lincoln) Asylum,' continues Dr Granville, ' he soon put me at my ease by conversing freely and unreservedly upon the subject which engrossed my attention at the time, and by frankly avowing himself the staunchest advocate of the plan, *as well as of the originator of it.'* It is plain that Dr Charlesworth could not make an ' originator ' out of Mr Hill!

"Once more, in 1850, at the dinner of the Provincial Medical and Surgical Association, at Hull, Dr Charlesworth declared publicly, that ' the real honour of first introducing the system was due to Mr Hill.' Thus far the testimony of Dr Charlesworth. ' Who will dare to desecrate his memory,' by asserting the above testimony is false ?

"But ' to whom does Dr Conolly award the praise of having led the way in that path which he himself has so honourably trodden ?' asks the *Lancet* and quotes the following passage from a letter of Dr Conolly's to Dr Charlesworth in reply :—' For I never can forget that it is to you that I and all of us are indebted for being roused to useful and benevolent exertion in behalf of the insane.' This does not state, however, that Dr Charlesworth roused him to the abolition of all restraint, but simply that he roused him and others to useful and benevolent exertion. May I also be permitted to quote a letter containing the sentiments of Dr Conolly on the abolition of re-straint :—

" ' 12 Old Burlington street, Jan. 6, 1851.

" ' Sir,—Please put my name down as a subscriber of one guinea to Mr Hill's testimonial. In advocating the claims of Dr Conolly, I have never overlooked those of Mr Hill as the originator of the non-restraint system in our Asylums. In proof that Dr Conolly himself does justice to Mr Hill's merits, Dr Conolly suggested to me, long ago, whether some portion of *his* subscription might not appropriately be devoted to the recognition of Mr Hill's claims. This, of course, could not be done.

" ' Yours faithfully,

" ' JOHN FORBES.'

" ' Rev. J. Daniel.' "

" ' And this will be the testimony of every one who shall honestly trace the history of the subject.' Dr Charlesworth mitigated, I abolished restraint: there is abundant honour due to Dr Charlesworth, but not the honour of the total abolition of all restraint. Why attempt to thrust that upon him after his death which he always disclaimed during his life? And why represent me as robbing the dead of his due, when all that I have written or spoken upon the subject was written and spoken *previously to his decease;* nor have I ever uttered a single syllable in disparagement of his efforts throughout a long series of years to mitigate the severity of restraint by every possible means. 'Suum cuique:' 'fiat justitia, ruat cœlum.'

" 'The Governors of the Lincoln Asylum,' says Sir Ed. Ff. Bromhead, ' never expressed a wish for the extinction of restraint; they never expected it; not one of them deemed it possible; *they did what they could in a proper direction—they mitigated evil.'*

" But the testimonial given to me as the originator of non-restraint, 'records the good-natured weakness of many, the personal feelings of some, the ignorance of others !' Strange, indeed! Let the author of this curious paragraph endeavour to prevail on ' the good-natured weakness of many, the personal feelings of some, and the ignorance of others,' to present *him* with a testimonial, on the ground of his being the originator of some great and novel improvement. Will he succeed? But who are the weak and ignorant subscribers to my testimonial? Can these terms indicate Mr Serjeant Adams, Sir J. Forbes, M.D.; Mr Gaskell, Commissioner in Lunacy; Dr Wingett, Dr Mackintosh, Dr Diamond, the Right Hon. R. A. Christopher, M.P.; Sir E. Bulwer Lytton, M.P.; Sir Henry Outram, M.D.; Rev. C. J. B. Smith, D.D.; Colonel Sibthorp, M.P.; Dr Nesbitt, and a whole host of similar names? What personal feelings can influence these eminent men towards a comparative stranger to many of them? True, the testimonial records the evidence of Dr Charlesworth and Sir Ed. Ff. Bromhead. Were they ' weak and ignorant men ?' But I leave the writer of this article, which is couched in such bitter and piercing terms against me, to his own reflections, convinced that he must see, if he have not the candour to own, the injustice of the attack which he has so unprovokedly made upon me in your columns.

"But I *failed* in carrying out my system. Did Dr Charlesworth say so? No; he dictated in part the following reply:—'It is true that in one single case since the above date, viz., in *April*, 1840, a patient was instrumentally restrained *for eighteen hours;* the circumstances solely imputable *to* a disorganised state of the staff of the attendants, and not to any failure in the system, *when* carried out in the manner laid down in my lecture, delivered June 21, 1838, and published in April, 1839. I still wait for a preclaimant to the system of totally abolishing instrumental restraint in the management of the insane.' The terms in which I announced the possibility of their abolition are as follows.—'In a properly constructed building, *with a sufficient number of suitable attendants,* restraint is never necessary, never justifiable, and always injurious in all cases of lunacy whatever.' If the attendants be in a state of disorganisation the system cannot be carried out. My own entry in the 'House-Surgeon's Journal,' 1840, March 29, explains the 'failure:' —'For want of proper attendants I have been obliged to sanction the personal restraint of a female patient who had previously passed more than two years without any such application.' . . 'This is the only instance of restraint which has occurred in the house for more than three successive years, and need not have happened now if the non-restraint system could have had fair play. It is to be hoped that a system which is now triumphantly progressing in other similar institutions will not be allowed to perish in its birthplace, strangled by withdrawing the means which I have always declared to be indispensable for its maintenance.' To quote this instance, then, as a 'failure,' is a manifest and wilful perversion of the fact, and a 'desecration of the memory of Dr Charlesworth,' who assisted me in defending myself against that imputation. Moreover, this reported 'failure,' occurred in April, 1840, and in January, 1841, Dr Charlesworth expressed a hope that the house-surgeon of that date would *succeed* in his object, *as Mr Hill has done in his own.* But, says the writer in the *Lancet*, 'the world will interpret it otherwise.' I leave the matter with all confidence to the world, to my contemporaries, and to posterity, and I feel no doubt that I shall receive ample justice. By all means let a memorial be raised, not by local subscriptions alone, but by national and cosmopolitan efforts; let his great and important services 'have a commensurate recognition,' but let not that memorial record that *he* was the originator of the non-restraint system, lest the very stone of which it is composed should cry out, 'Is there not a lie in my right hand?'

    " I have the honour to be,

        " Your faithful and obedient servant,

            " ROBERT GARDINER HILL, F.S.A.

           " One of the Visitors of the Lincolnshire

               " County Lunatic Asylum.

" Eastgate House, Lincoln,

    " Nov. 12, 1853."

From the *Medical Circular*, November 23, 1853.—

      " MR HILL AND THE 'LANCET.'

        " Dundee Royal Asylum, 8th, Nov., 1853.

" DEAR SIR,—The unwarrantable attack made upon your professional character by the Editor of the *Lancet*, in his leading article of the 5th instant, and the audacious insinuations which he has thrown out regarding the motives actuating the contributors to your late testimonial, have caused me some astonishment, but much more regret, that so much special pleading and detraction, with a view to under-estimate the amount and originality of your labours on behalf of the insane, should have emanated from so influential a quarter. My present object in writing you is simply to express that regret. I do not, as yet, know how the criticism of the *Lancet* is regarded by that section of the profession engaged in treating insanity as their speciality, and who may be supposed to be well-informed upon the facts of the case, but I feel it to be due to you to lose no time in assuring you that, as *one* member of that body, I regard the criticism in question as being lamentably unjust and partial, and as being a laboured attempt wilfully to hide, misinterpret, and ignore the more important facts of the matter at issue.

" The points of difference in the claims and merits of Dr Charlesworth and yourself, are clear and decided; and I cannot conceive how an impartial on-looker can form any other judgment than that arrived at by the contributors to your testimonial. If the system of treatment by the *total abolition* of restraint were really a boon, blessing, and discovery, then the question *was* and *is* — Who was its author ? The answer *was* and *is* — The man who first advanced the proposition that the use of mechanical restraints is injurious and ought to be dispensed with in the treatment of all cases of insanity whatever. Now *you* were undoubtedly that man :—and immediately upon your announcement of that fact, there existed *two* systems or methods of treatment where *one* existed before. Non-restraint, as a fact of universal application in the treatment of insanity was, up to this time, unheard of. Thus, the impartial history of these two systems will record that the *one* was inaugurated by Pinel, in 1792, the *other* by yourself, in 1837. The merit of Dr Charlesworth consisted in reiterating the teaching, and imitating the practice of Pinel, which was to dispense with restraint *as much as possible*. In pursuing this laudable course he had many worthy and successful contemporaries who were working in the same field of benevolence, and who advocated the claims of the lunatic in numerous interesting and powerful appeals to the public. Esquirol, Conolly, and Browne were among the more distinguished of his fellow-labourers. But the *total abolition of restraint* was not yet advocated. It was your undoubted merit to have been the first to affirm its practicability and necessity. Upon this point hinges the whole question. Dr Charlesworth clearly limited himself to the propriety of the *modified use* of restraint. You, on the other hand, inculcated its uncompromising and *entire disuse*. Dr Charlesworth's own unambiguous words confirm this view of the matter. With these facts before us, when I and others took in hand to present the author of the non-restraint method with a testimonial, we had no doubt whatever in regard to the identity of the man who was entitled to our approbation; nor can I understand how any man can find difficulty or doubt in forming the same judgment, provided he simply brings to the inquiry an honest and sincere desire to give a just and true award. In attaining our object, we certainly could not so far stultify ourselves as to give our offering to the man who, previously to your own announcement, had uniformly taught and practised the system to which your own was opposed. Nevertheless, the editor of the *Lancet* would seem to argue that this was our proper course, when he grounds the claims of Dr Charlesworth upon the fact that his labours were preparatory and introductory to your own, and proceeds to force the inference that Dr Charlesworth had already conceived and was influenced by the idea which you were the first to utter. There is no evidence whatever to justify such a decision. It is clearly a gratuitous assumption, and cannot bear the gaze of an impartial inquirer. No doubt every man who favours the world with a new idea is indebted to others for preparing the way for its development,

U

but our thanks are not on that account confined to the authors of these precursory or preparatory achievements. We never hesitate to applaud the man who gives to the labours of his predecessors a new and more extended application. James Watt is regarded as the author of the steam-engine, and as such our praise and gratitude are lavished upon him; nevertheless, he was preceded in his labours, and, in the sense of the editor of the *Lancet*, anticipated or forestalled by Brancas, of Rome; the Marquis of Worcester; Salomon de Caus, the mad inmate of the Bicêtre; Captain Savary; and Thomas Newcomen. All these labourers paved the way for James Watt, but his own crowning idea gave a new aspect to the whole machine, and the world has allowed him to claim it as his own.

"In this matter of non-restraint, I and others who contributed to your testimonial desired to congratulate and applaud the man who had carried progress and improvement to a limit which it had never before attained, and who had made that progress the basis of a system designed to take the place of the one then practised. There could be no mistake that you were the author of the novelty in question; nevertheless, the editor of the *Lancet*, in his recent criticism, characterizes the conduct of those who recognised the value of your services, as indicative either of ' good-natured weakness' or 'ignorance.' Our conduct admits, however, of another interpretation; and you may rest assured that whoever desires to arrive at a deliberate and dispassionate judgment upon the nature of your merits and right, will condemn this critique of the *Lancet* as being defective, exaggerated, partial, and disingenuous; in fact, as being an unworthy attempt to injure a reputation laudably acquired and widely recognised.

"I am, dear Sir, faithfully yours,

"T. T. Wingett, M.D.

"R. Gardiner Hill, Esq., Lincoln."

From the *Lancet*, December 3, 1853.

" Sir,—Our attention has been directed to an article in a scurrilous medical print, in which the committee for raising a memorial to the late Dr Charlesworth are indirectly charged with having paid for a leading article in the *Lancet*, of the 5th inst., with a view to raise subscriptions for that memorial.

" Had such a base and unfounded charge been confined to the pages of the low print in question, it might have been safely treated with contempt ; but, as it has been industriously circulated by means of advertisements in various papers, I trust you will allow us to give the charge our most unqualified and indignant denial.

" We are, Sir, your obedient servants,
" WM. PIERCE, A.M.
" JAMES SNOW, F.R.C.S. Eng.
Hon. Secs. to the Charlesworth Memorial Committee."
" Lincoln, Nov. 28th, 1853."

1853, *December 9.* — *Stamford Mercury.* — " BRIBING THE ' LANCET.'—An advertisement, in the form of a letter, addressed to the Editor of the *Lancet*, signed W. M. Pierce, A.M., and James Snow, F.R.C.S.E., having appeared in the *Stamford Mercury*, repudiating any attempt to bribe the *Lancet*, in connection with raising subscriptions for the ' Charlesworth Testimonial,' a letter will be published in the *Medical Circular* for Dec. 14, from the Rev. W. M. Pierce, to the Editor of that journal (the *Medical Circular*) offering to pay for the insertion of an article prejudicial to Mr Gardiner Hill, and in advocacy of the Charlesworth Testimonial Fund.

" Medical Circular Office, 128 Strand,
" Dec. 5, 1853."

1853, *December* 14.—The *Medical Circular*, Leading Article :—

"BRIBING THE 'LANCET.'

" Our readers will recollect that a few weeks since the *Lancet* published a leading article, in which it unfairly attempted to depreciate the claim of Mr Robert Gardiner Hill to be considered the originator of the 'non-restraint' system of treatment in lunacy, and subsequently refused that gentleman the right of exposing the deceptive arguments, and of defending himself against the slanderous aspersions that had been cast upon his character. Indignant at the mingled injustice and meanness of this conduct, we published in the *Medical Circular* the reply of Mr Hill, with some editorial observations, explaining the facts of the question and supporting his claim.

" That the course we pursued stung the conductors of the *Lancet*, and rebuked the individuals who secretly stimulated its hostility to Mr Robert Gardiner Hill, is not surprising, but we must confess that we hardly expected that the *Lancet* would be foolish enough to assail us with the elegant epistle it published in a recent number, duly authenticated with the illustrious names of 'Wm. Pierce' and 'James Snow.' We give a transcript, verbatim, of this literary curiosity :—

" 'TO THE EDITOR OF THE 'LANCET.'

" ' Sir,—Our attention has been directed to an article in an obscure medical print, in which the Committee for raising a Memorial to the late Dr Charlesworth are indirectly charged with having paid for a leading article in the *Lancet* of the 5th inst., with a view to raise subscriptions for that memorial.

" ' Had such a base and unfounded charge been confined to the pages of the low print in question, it might have been safely treated with contempt; but, as it has been industriously circulated, by means of advertisements in various papers, I trust you will allow us to give the charge our most unqualified and indignant denial.

"‘ We are, Sir, your obedient servants,

"‘ Wm. Pierce, A.M.,⠀⠀ ⎱Honorary

"‘ James Snow, F.R.C.S.E.,⎰Secretaries

"‘ to the Charlesworth Memorial Committee.

"‘ Lincoln, November 28, 1853.'

"We confidently believe that neither Mr Pierce nor Mr Snow wrote this letter, but that it was concocted in the *Lancet* office for the purpose of puffing that journal, which is rapidly and deservedly decaying both in credit and circulation. We believe so, because the language applied to us is exactly that which the vulgar genius of the *Lancet* is in the habit of using in connexion with the name of the *Medical Circular;* and because, too, the Rev. Mr Pierce, if he be a sane man, never could have been so indiscreet as voluntarily to indite such a letter while retaining a recollection of one he had previously written to ourselves.

"It is distinctly asserted that we have charged the *Lancet* with receiving a bribe for its leading article. We cannot deny what every literary medical man knows to be true, that the *Lancet* is pre-eminently a venal paper; but we are puzzled to understand what good reason the *Lancet* had for seeking for and publishing the contemptible certificate of character which we have quoted. The article to which the letter refers runs thus :

"‘ Two months ago, *a certain gentleman* sent to us for publication a series of printed documents, containing a letter and appendices, which had been put into circulation more than two years prior to our being favoured with the communication, and which, had they been accepted, would have occupied together about a dozen columns of the *Medical Circular*, and in a letter accompanying the documents offered to *pay* US for the accorded privilege of publication. On perusing the papers we discovered that they disclosed an elaborate attempt to expose and degrade the character of Mr Robert Gardiner Hill, Mayor of Lincoln ; we therefore disdained to accept the paltry bribe, and resolved that our pages should never be made the medium of purchased vituperation. Our advertising sheet is the proper place for a marketable transaction.'—*Medical Circular*, No. 45, p. 354.

" Our charge is, that a certain gentleman offered to pay US—not the *Lancet*—and we observed, at the end of the following paragraph—' We should like to know how much has been paid into its (the *Lancet's*) treasury, in requital of the slavish service it has rendered to the miserable faction whose cause it espouses.' Every sensible man will see that this was no charge at all, but a question, arising out of a very natural and obvious inference; and will suspect, with us, that the *Lancet*, painfully conscious of many offences of this shameful kind, was glad of the opportunity of making a merit of one possibly exceptional act of public virtue. The letter then is a mere Bobadil brag ;—a farcical piece of bluster, assumed to screen a career of habitual corruption.

" This impudent letter, our readers will remark, is signed by a WM. PIERCE, who is a reverend gentleman of the church, and, for his benefit and for ours, we append another epistle, rather more oily in its style, signed by the *same gentleman* :

" ' TO THE EDITOR OF THE ' MEDICAL CIRCULAR.'

" ' Sir,—My attention has been directed to a paper in your last publication, and I am induced to send you a copy of a letter I felt it right to publish some time since upon a subject incidentally introduced into that paper (a biographical sketch of Mr G. Hill), and you will oblige me if you can find space for it in your next *Medical Circular*.

" ' *Allow me to add, that if articles of* THIS KIND *are required to be* PAID FOR, *I shall cheerfully meet your demand.*

" ' I have no intention to re-open a controversy which I feel is for ever settled, and still less any desire to deprive the late House-Surgeon of the Lincoln Lunatic Asylum of his fair share of praise and honour in connexion with the subject of my letter, but I feel that the cause of truth, and the memory of Dr Charlesworth, require this at my hands.

" ' I take the liberty, also, to enclose an extract from a lecture lately delivered by Dr Connolly, on the subject of the Treatment of the Insane; likewise a short memoir of the late Dr Charlesworth, which appeared in the *Lancet,* with a list of subscriptions for the purpose of placing a statue of Dr Charlesworth in the grounds of the Lincoln Lunatic Asylum.

" ' I shall be in London for a few days, when a line will find me if addressed to No. 43 Tredegar square, Bow road.

" ' I have the honour to be your obedient servant,

" ' W. M. PIERCE.

" ' West Ashby, Horncastle,

" ' Sept. 12, 1853.' "

" Can the Rev. Wm. Pierce hold up his head in Lincoln after the publication of this letter ? Is HE the man to be ' *indignant*' at a charge of bribery ? Did HE never offer to pay a journalist for the insertion of articles, ' with a view to raise subscriptions for Dr Charlesworth's Memorial;' or even for a less creditable object ? Publish this letter, Mr Pierce, of which, being signed with your own name, you ought not to be ashamed.

" We can prove that this is not the first time that this reverend gentleman has performed before the world in a similar questionable character.

" We now leave the Rev. Wm. M. Pierce and the Charlesworth Testimonial to the people of Lincoln, who, we trust, will deal with both according to their deserts.

"As for the *Lancet,* it has already fallen too low to sink to deeper ignominy."

From the *Medical Circular,* February 15, 1854.—
Leading Article.

THE NON-RESTRAINT SYSTEM OF TREATMENT IN LUNACY.

"In another column we publish a letter from Dr Leeuwen, addressed to Mr Robert Gardiner Hill, in which the claim of this gentleman to be considered the originator of the non-restraint system of treatment in lunacy is ably defended. It must be agreeable to the feelings of Mr Hill to find his cause supported by an independent witness—that witness a foreign physician, thoroughly acquainted with the documents that have been published on the subject, exempt from partialities, and aloof from the petty personal jealousies that have in this country perverted the simplicity of spontaneous testimony, and either obscured or falsified the truth, though written in undeniable official records. The letter of Dr Leeuwen is a triumphant reply to the intricate mesh of misrepresentation that has been fabricated in Lincoln, retailed from the *Lancet* office in London, and assiduously distributed among the credulous, the envious, and the ignorant.

"The period is coming round when the Board of Governors of the Lincoln Asylum will be required to publish their Annual Report, and, as a matter of course, its framers will feel it their duty to notice, in complimentary terms, the long and valuable services of the late Dr Charlesworth as Visiting Physician to their Institution. We acknowledge the merit and usefulness of this gentleman's labours ; we give him credit for benevolence, truthfulness, and an ardent sympathy with suffering ; we admit his acuteness, his zeal, his perseverance and habits of business ; more than all, we are glad to recognise the prompt, cordial, and steady support he extended to Mr Hill during the time this gentleman was engaged in carrying out his " *bold conception* " of the possibility of the entire abolition of restraint at the Lincoln Asylum. Dr Charlesworth is entitled to the praise of having mitigated *the system of coercion* as much, probably more, than any other individual in this country, and on this account alone his name deserves to be printed in red letters in the Lincoln Calendar; but will any man venture to record more than this to his honour? Will any scribe, after the exposition of the case in our pages be bold enough to assert that Dr Charlesworth is entitled to the praise rightfully belonging to Mr Hill, of being the originator of the principle of non-restraint in the treatment of Lunacy?

" That there may be no mistake on this subject we will quote paragraphs from the Reports of the Lincoln Asylum for the years 1837 and 1838. The first says :

" ' The present House-Surgeon has expressed *his own* belief, founded on experience in this house, that it may be possible to conduct an institution for the insane without having recourse to the employment of any instruments of restraint whatsoever.'—*Extract from the Thirteenth Annual Report, April* 12, 1837.

" The second contains this sentence :—

" ' The *bold conception* of pushing the mitigation of restraint to the extent of actually and formally abolishing the practice, *mentioned in the last Report as due to Mr Hill,* the House- Surgeon, seems to be justified by the following abstract of a statistical table, showing the rapid advance of the abatement of restraints in this Asylum, under an improved construction of the building, night-watching, and attentive supervision. We may venture to affirm that this is the first frank statement of the common practice of restraints hitherto laid before a British public.'—*Extracted from the Fourteenth Annual Report, March* 1838.

" Let it be remembered that *these Reports were written by Dr Charlesworth!* He received the thanks of the Board for his labours;—these documents must be therefore regarded as expressing his calm and deliberate judgment on the claims of Mr Hill. Dr Charlesworth, in the Report for 1837, distinctly states that Mr Hill has expressed *his own* belief—not Dr Charlesworth's—and in the Report for 1838, credits him with the ' bold conception' of a definitive abolition of the practice of restraint.

" In the latter year Mr Hill delivered, at Lincoln, his well-known ' Lecture on the Management of Lunatic Asylums,' in which he styles the mode of treatment in force on his acceptance of office, as the ' *old principle*,' claims the credit of announcing a ' *new system*,' describes it as ' *my theory*,' and in one part, in which he relates the difficulties he encountered, the laborious attention he gave to the cases, and the gradual growth of his conviction that the use of restraints might be abolished, he says—*at length* I felt convinced there was little occasion for the restraint, and resolved WITHIN MYSELF *to discontinue its use altogether*.' (Page 48.) Here was the expression of a *secret* resolution, arrived at after long experience and much reflection,—not, be it remarked, the adoption of the views, wishes, or instructions of any other man. When we inform our readers that Dr Charlesworth read and revised this lecture previous to its publication, he must be considered to have concurred in the claims of Mr Hill.

" Moreover, when Mr Hill was subsequently assailed in the *Lancet*, and his claims disputed, he replied in a letter containing this sentence:—' The acrimonious attacks to which my prominent position as the originator of the total abolition of instrumental restraint in lunacy has exposed me from its opponents, make it necessary that I should resort to this measure of *self*-protection, from irresponsible antagonists.' This letter was revised by Dr Charlesworth prior to publication, and the word *self*, printed in italics in the quotation, was added by Dr Charlesworth, thus individualising, *by his own act,* Mr Hill as the only person to whom the credit of *originating* the new system could possibly apply.

" Finally, at the Anniversary Meeting of the Provincial Association held at Hull, Dr Charlesworth said emphatically, ' The *real honour* of *first* introducing the system is due to Mr Hill ! ' No testimony can be more direct, unqualified, or explicit. Will any individual, after these repeated declarations, dare to snatch the laurels from the head of Mr Hill to crown therewith the statue of Dr Charlesworth ? The memory of Dr Charlesworth will resent the insult to his honour. Who will be at the pains, after his death, to prove him, during life, insincere, sinister, and false?

" The forthcoming Annual Report will be drawn up by Sir E. Ff. Bromhead, who, from having been once the friend, is now the opponent of Mr Hill. Lest this gentleman should be tempted by partizanship to deviate from the letter of the written record, we beg to remind him of his antecedent opinions. Sir E. Ff. Bromhead was Vice-President of the Lincoln Asylum when those Reports, *drawn up by Dr Charlesworth,* to which we have already alluded, were presented and published; he also occupied the chair at the Mechanics' Institution when Mr Hill delivered his lecture, in which he boldly claimed to be the ' *originator* ' of the ' *new system.*' He heard the quotations from the Reports read by Mr Hill, and he formally approved every statement contained in the lecture by moving a vote of thanks to this gentleman.

" Further than this, on the publication of this lecture he *reviewed* it in the pages of the *Lincoln Standard* of the 15th of May, 1839, and Dr Charlesworth *revised* his review. In the course of the article we find these sentences :—

" ' Mr Hill had for some time successfully carried into operation at our Asylum the total abolition of all restraint and all severity before he presented himself to the public

as the deliverer of a Lecture on the subject . . . . . In this
lecture, Mr Hill exhibits a frightful picture of the ancient
abuses universally inflicted on the insane, until the benevolent Pinel made an inroad on this domain of cruelty.
He *began* what Mr Hill *completed* . . . . At Lincoln the boards
resolutely set about to ameliorate the treatment, and have
confirmed the remark, ' were every one to see the whole
effects, mediate and immediate, present and remote, even of
trifling acts of good or evil, his mind would, on many occasions, be filled with delight or remorse.' *The Governors never
expressed a wish for the extinction of restraints; they never
expected it; not one of them deemed it possible;* they did all the
good they could in a proper direction, they mitigated evil.
They elected an honest, firm, sensible, and benignant medical
man as a resident officer, they placed every possible facility
in his way: and this honest and good man found himself
landed triumphantly on an unhoped-for territory. He had
much to struggle with;—the character of visionary humanity
—the underplot of reluctant servants, who found every step
in his progress a trespass on their own repose; and it may be
considered most fortunate for mankind that no unlucky
apropos fatal accident blasted the plan for ever.'

" This is strong language, but Sir Edward Ff. Bromhead
has, accorded to Mr Hill, if possible, even more distinct
and emphatic praise. He has expressly denominated the
system of non-restraint ' HIS SYSTEM !' When Mr Hill
was a candidate for the office of Superintendent of the
Bodmin Asylum, Sir E. Ff. Bromhead addressed a letter-
testimonial in his favour to the Chairman of the Board,
wherein we find it stated:

" ' It is most honourable to him, that when I was in the
chair on Mr Hill's retiring from office, the vote of regret
for his loss, and thanks for his services, passed the Board
unanimously, though the opponents of HIS *system of throwing
aside the strait-waistcoat and chains,* were then present.

Most unhappily, this great improvement has been deemed a *rebuke to the practice of Mr Hill's predecessors*, and the practice of other houses, and has drawn much acrimonious exaggeration and even mis-statement against the practice, and finally, as might be expected, some hostility to the AUTHOR, from the party favourable to instrumental restraint and their friends.'

"Here Sir Ff. Bromhead not only calls him the AUTHOR of the new system, but goes so far as to say, that unhappily it has been deemed 'a rebuke to the practice of Mr Hill's predecessors,' thus unequivocally showing that Mr Hill's predecessors neither practised nor recognised the system, and that the credit of it is entirely his own.

"We recall these matters to the memory of Sir E. Ff. Bromhead in order that, should he be induced, from partiality, friendship, or any other motive, to ascribe to the late Dr Charlesworth credit that belongs to another, he may not have the excuse of forgetfulness or misconception. If, in the performance of his duty of bringing up this Report, he should be assisted by his coadjutors, Mr Snow and Mr Throsby, we hope that Sir Edward Ff. Bromhead will have the honesty and manliness to expunge from the Record any expressions inconsistent with the statements in the Reports for 1837 and 1838, the express declarations of Dr Charlesworth, his own written opinions, and the plain unvarnished truth of the question. We ask this in justice to Mr Hill — nay, more, in justice to the honoured memory of Dr Charlesworth.

"Inasmuch, however, as the new Board cannot possibly either appreciate the feelings of the Boards of 1837 and 1838, or have a personal knowledge of the facts on which those Boards grounded their opinions, we cannot believe that it will be guilty of the presumption of attempting to reverse the decisions recorded in previous Reports; nor can we suppose that Sir E. Ff. Bromhead, who is a man of good sense and punctilious honour, will, after due reflection, seek to accomplish such a preposterous and unjustifiable design."

From the *Medical Circular*, February 15, 1854:—

"THE NON-RESTRAINT SYSTEM.

"TO THE EDITOR OF THE 'MEDICAL CIRCULAR.'

" Sir,—The accompanying letter contains the *impartial judgment* of an *unprejudiced* and *distinguished foreigner*. Will you oblige me by giving it insertion in the next number of your valuable journal ?

" Your obliged servant,

"ROBERT GARDINER HILL.

" Eastgate House, Lincoln,
  " Feb. 7, 1854."

(*Copy.*)

" ' Jersey, January 21, 1854.

" ' My dear Sir,—Although personally unknown to you, I cannot help expressing to you my great surprise and sorrow about the personal and inimical way towards you, in which it seems that the late Dr Charlesworth's merits must be vindicated.

" ' When two years ago I wrote a rather long paper on the Non-Restraint System for the Dutch journal, *Nederlandich Lancet,* I had to derive all my information from the Reports on the State of the Lincoln Lunatic Asylum, and in the Thirteenth Annual Report [written by Dr CHARLES-WORTH, and signed W. M. PIERCE, *vide* Minute Book, April 12, 1837], page 5, I made your first acquaintance as the *owner of the belief,* founded on experience in the Lincoln Asylum, 'that it may be possible to conduct an Institution for the Insane without having recourse to the employment of any instruments of restraint whatever.' For in plain and express terms I read these words,—' The present House-Surgeon has expressed his *own* belief that it may be possible . . &c.' In the following Annual Report (1838), [written and signed by E. P. CHARLESWORTH, *vide* Minute Book, March 19, 1838], I read, 'The bold conception of pushing the mitigation of restraint to the extent of actually and formally abolishing the practice, mentioned in the last Report as *due* to Mr Hill, the House-Surgeon, seems to be justified, &c.' Nothing could be plainer and clearer, and more exclusive of anybody else being the *original owner of the bold conception* mentioned, and in my Dutch paper nobody but Mr HILL was mentioned as the originator of the Non-Restraint System. After a relation of the introduction of this system in the Lincoln Asylum, I gave in the same way, *i. e.* by extracts from the Hanwell Reports, the history of it in Hanwell; and in my critical remarks on both Asylums at the end of my paper I could not help giving the preference, as to the different methods in which the Non-Restraint System was carried out in Lincoln and Hanwell, to the principles and practice pursued by Dr Conolly, as I could not either agree with the *simultaneous abolition* of all seclusion of the insane for a few hours in a single room, or with the rejecting of a proper out-door classification, &c., which the Board of Managers of the Lincoln Asylum thought better to dispense with altogether. I was happy to find, in the 'Further Report of the Commissioners in Lunacy of 1847,' that I was not the only one who thought that the Board of Managers of the Lincoln Asylum carried things too far, and the uncourteous answer of the Governors of the Lincoln Lunatic Asylum to the Visiting Commissioners in Lunacy, contained in Appendix (H) of the 'Further Report, pages 363—378,' seemed to justify my fear that there was some false ambition among the Governors of the Lincoln Lunatic Asylum of aiming at too much. If, therefore, as to the abolition of restraint, I thought the Lincoln Asylum deserved all the honour of the priority before other Asylums, yet I then did not at all think

the Lincoln Asylum to be such a *model* or *perfect example* as
its Board of Governors seemed to think it. And, in fact, all
reports of foreigners who visited it—for instance, of Dr
Schlemm, who published a Report on British Asylums in
1848, gave a similar unfavourable opinion of the Lincoln
Asylum. I mentioned, however, in my pamphlet,
that the less fortunate development of the Lincoln
Asylum, as a kind of model, ought not to reflect any discredit
upon the non-restraint system, nor upon Mr Hill, because Mr
Hill had left the Asylum as Resident Medical Superintendent
in 1840, and the non-restraint system had proved most
beneficial wherever it was introduced.

" ' Since I wrote my Dutch paper, in 1852, I have, in
1853, been engaged in making a French Report to the
States of Jersey on some French Asylums which I visited
in January and February, 1853, and I have thought it my
duty to vindicate, in this report, the honour of the English
system against the wrong and unjust critiques of the French
authors. In trying to do so, not by robbing the French of
their merits, but by testing the results of the French system
in comparison with the results of the English, I have again
consulted the original sources for the history of the non-
restraint system, and I did this with the greater interest, as
I found that the death of Dr Charlesworth had excited a
controversy on its authorship. Again, I have not been able
to make out that Dr Charlesworth was the *original owner of
the bold conception*, unless the managers have made statements
which they knew to be lies in the Annual Reports of the
Lincoln Asylum in 1837 and 1838. In consequence of my
renewed inquiry, I have therefore stated again in my French
Report that Mr Hill was the originator of the Non-Restraint
System; for to say that I suppose the Board of Managers
of Lincoln Asylum in 1837 and 1838 to have been liars
would be discourteous and what I do not believe.

" ' You can, therefore, my dear sir, fancy how surprised

and sorry I am that some other people now try to rob you of an honour, of which the reports of Lincoln Asylum prove you to be the *owner*. I am glad, however, to see that they dig their own grave with this hard work : the personal attacks against you, as no assertions can undo what the Reports of Lincoln have stated to be the truth, prove the weakness and wickedness of your enemies. Besides this personal enmity against you, they seem not to know much of the history of lunacy in England, as they overlook entirely all the claims which the celebrated family of the Tukes, in the York Friends' Retreat, no doubt possess, of having introduced Pinel's great reformation from France into England. The claims of Dr Charlesworth are no doubt great, and he is worthy of a monument, but his claims are, in my opinion, none other but those due to the Tukes, who (if it is a claim to have imitated the example of Pinel) have also the claim of priority over Dr Charlesworth. Dr Charlesworth, however, may have done more in elaborating and in writing down principles—this is possible—and far from me be the desire of depriving him of his merits!

" Now, Sir, I will end. Allow me to add only my modest opinion on the course which I advise you to take in a moral struggle which cannot but have embittered temporarily your happiness and that of your family and friends. Let them all say what they like against you, and do not trouble yourself about it any more. What is honour and glory after our death ? This prospect seems to me too empty to fight much for. Let them rather rob you of your future glory than your present happiness. Enjoy the present honour which your enemies give you in giving them so much trouble for that *bold conception* which the Lincoln Reports, as long as they last, will always tell in plain words, that *you are the original owner of;* let your enemies lend this ownership to their friend Dr Charlesworth, who seems to want it very much in their eyes.

x

"Is not the dismissal of Mr Gay from the Royal Free Hospital a shameful fact? What an honour, almost, it begins to be, to be blamed by the leaders of the *Lancet!* I am only sorry that Dr Forbes Winslow has admitted the last article against you in his valuable journal. But I am sure he is too honourable a man, and a too impartial inquirer after truth if he will at once cast his eyes into the Reports of the Lincoln Asylum, not to acknowledge what is stated there so plainly, *that the bold conception of abolishing all instrumental restraint is due to Mr Hill,* because he first expressed his *own* belief about it, when it was yet prudently looked upon with disbelief by every one else but him;—because Mr Hill spent three hours daily for thirty-eight out of forty successive days among the insane, only for the purpose of testing the system on the disorderly patients; and in fact, because all the troubles and merits of the immediate wear and tear of a lunatic Asylum strike only the resident medical officers, but not the visiting physicians.

"Forgive me if I have been rather long. Whenever I find an opportunity of visiting Lincoln, I hope to make your acquaintance.

"Believe me, my dear Sir,

"Yours very Sincerely,

"D. H. VAN LEEUWEN,

"Late one of the Resident Physicians to the Provincial Asylum, Meerenberg, Noord, Holland.

"To Robert Gardiner Hill, Esq., F.S.A.

"Eastgate House, Lincoln."

(Appendix F.)

Opinions of the 'Lancet' from 1840 to 1852 in favour of the Author's claims. Testimony of Richard Mason, Esq., late Town Clerk of Lincoln and a Governor of the Lincoln Lunatic Asylum.

From the *Lancet*, December 1840, p. 377.—Leading Article.

" If Bethlem, St Luke, and several other large Asylums, have remained stationary, or have retrograded, the Quaker's Asylum, some private establishments, the Scotch Asylums, the Lincoln Asylum, and latterly, Hanwell, have persevered, and have carried out the rational system to an extent which had not before been deemed possible. Mr HILL and Dr CHARLESWORTH first declared themselves the advocates of the ' *non-restraint system,*' which appears destined to form an epoch in the treatment of the disease.

" The term ' non-restraint,' we may remark, is not literally correct; for, when the system is most rigidly carried out, the patient is *confined* to the Asylum, and in many cases to his room. But this confinement is not felt like fetters; it is less degrading, irritating, and exasperating than ligatures on the limbs. The restraint is little more severe than the voluntary confinement of servants to the house, or of workmen to their daily task. The violent, raving maniac has, however, necessarily to submit to further restraint; the keepers' arms are also called into action, and have to supply the place of the strait waistcoat, straps, and chains. The only question that admits of controversy, is, whether, when coercion of some kind is required, and applied by all parties, bands, instrumental restraint, and mechanical advantages should be altogether discarded, and replaced by the force of the keepers' hands and arms? Under which treatment does the patient suffer least, and has he the best chance of a speedy recovery, the exclusive ' keeper restraint' system, or the mixed treatment, in which instrumental restraint is partially employed? and, if it should turn out that the advantages are pretty equally balanced, or that they preponderate in favour of occasional mechanical restraint, are not the liabilities to the excessive application of instruments, adequate reasons for foregoing the use of an agent that may be dispensed with, and is likely to be abused by the keepers, at least in large Asylums ? "

From the ' LANCET,' *October* 26, 1850.—Leading Article.

" THE treatment of lunatics and the management of Asylums have recently occupied much attention in England, as also on the Continent, and in America. France took the lead in this philanthropic movement, about the end of last century, at which period M. Tenon visited London, in order to obtain information respecting the system pursued at Bethlem and other lunatic hospitals. On his return to Paris, in 1786, as a first step in the right direction, the French Government withdrew the insane from the Hôtel Dieu, to which they had been previously consigned, in order to place them in Asylums specially erected for their reception. Subsequently, Pinel, Esquirol, and other eminent persons, carried forward the good work thus happily begun by Tenon, whereby a great impetus was given to the cause of suffering humanity throughout the civilized world.

" For many years England lagged very much behind in this movement: and at Bethlem, and other hospitals, the

Parliamentary Inquiry, instituted in 1815, disclosed atrocities which now seem scarcely credible. However, the recent labours of Gardiner Hill, Conolly, and other distinguished individuals, have altogether abolished the coercive treatment formerly pursued towards the afflicted lunatic in this country; and now, without being carried away by national vanity, we may safely assert, that England has far surpassed her continental neighbours in the treatment of the insane, especially in reference to the great question of mechanical personal restraint.' "

From the *Lancet*, November 8, 1851.

" TESTIMONIAL TO ROBERT GARDINER HILL, ESQ.

" On the evening of Wednesday week last the splendid testimonial, purchased by subscription, by the friends of Mr Robert Gardiner Hill, the originator of the non-restraint system, was presented at a banquet, held at the Great Northern Hotel, in Lincoln, to that gentleman, in the presence of a numerous and fashionable circle of ladies and gentlemen, gathered together to do honour to the occasion. The testimonial consisted of a handsome silver centre-piece. The Mayor, in presenting the testimonial, spoke in flattering terms of the great services rendered to the humane cause of non-restraint in cases of lunacy. He stated that the testimonial had been subscribed to not only by the personal friends of Mr Hill, but by a number of the medical profession, scattered over England, in justice to Mr Hill. Mr Hill returned thanks in a speech of much eloquence and ability. Several other gentlemen addressed the meeting, which was respectably and numerously attended. The inscription on the testimonial is as follows :—

" ' Presented, together with a silver tea-service, to Robert Gardiner Hill, Esq., M.R.C.S. Eng., author and originator of the Total Abolition of Restraint in the

Treatment of the Insane, now commonly called the "Non-Restraint System," by a number of subscribers, medical and general, from all parts of the kingdom, in token of their admiration of the talent which could devise, and the energy and patient perseverance which, despite of prejudice, opposition, and jealousy, could carry out a system fraught with results so eminently beneficial to mankind.'

"This is engraven on one side of the centre-piece: on the other side is inscribed the following extracts from the Annual Reports of the Lincoln Lunatic Asylum:

"'It was Mr Hill who had the courage to broach the original and invaluable idea that the use of instruments might be wholly dispensed with.'—Sir E. Ff. BROMHEAD, Bart., Vice-President of the Lincoln Asylum.

"'The real honour belonged to Mr Hill, of the Lincoln Asylum.'—Dr CHARLESWORTH."

From the *Lancet*, November 20, 1852.—Leading Article:

"In the columns for news is inserted a paragraph from the *Stamford Mercury*, which contains an account of the election of Mr Robert Gardiner Hill as Mayor of Lincoln. We refer to this election with feelings of much satisfaction, because it is a tribute of respect to a most worthy member of our profession. For many years the name of Mr Hill has been identified with the humane treatment of lunatics. Like other upholders of this system he has met with many difficulties and much opposition : he has persevered and been successful. Many will echo the sentiments which fell from Mr Harvey, the seconder of his nomination."

From the *Lancet*, November 20, 1852 :—

"ELECTION OF MR ROBERT GARDINER HILL AS MAYOR OF LINCOLN.—At the last meeting of the Corporation Mr Carline rose to propose a successor to the gentleman who was about to retire from the mayoralty, and who, he was certain, would receive the thanks of the council, and the sincere approval of the citizens, for the high integrity and great ability which had marked his discharge of the multiform and onerous duties of the chief magistracy. In naming Mr Hill for the next year, he would admit that that gentleman did not possess those qualifications, the fruit of ripened experience in civic matters, which distinguished the retiring mayor; but Mr Hill was eminent for his calmness, deliberation, and firmness, and these qualities, united with the great common sense which he was well known to possess, would enable him to perform the duties of the office with credit and dignity, and to the entire satisfaction of the citizens. (Cheers.)

"Mr Harvey seconded the nomination. A private friendship of twenty-five years, and twelve years' connexion with Mr Hill in business, had afforded him ample opportunity of satisfying himself of the possession by Mr Hill of those excellent qualities which won and preserved esteem, and which were a guarantee that the duties linked with the honour about to be conferred upon him would be discharged with a diligence and integrity that could not be surpassed. (Cheers.) Years since it had been remarked by one well acquainted with human nature, that he knew no one less satisfied with the mere performance of his duty than Mr Hill; and that feature, which was the characteristic of the young man, was not less distinct in the mature man. That Mr Hill was honoured and esteemed by the citizens of Lincoln had been demonstrated upon several occasions, and the present unanimous intention to confer upon him the highest honour it was in the power of the city to bestow was another proof of the estimation in which he was held. But the name of Mr Hill was known and respected far beyond the city in which his patient diligence and enduring faith, in contention with a tide of difficulties that would have overwhelmed many men, enabled him to work out and demonstrate a great and philanthropical problem, and convert the system of treatment of the insane from one of barbarity to one of humanity and kindness. Humanity, sooner or later, had its lasting reward, and he (Mr Harvey) begged leave to express his calm confidence that the time would arrive when society would pay Mr Hill the debt of acknowledgment due to him as a great benefactor of mankind, by recording his name in history with the names of the great philanthropists who would be honoured and revered as long as the land's language lasted. (Cheers.)

"No other gentleman being proposed, the Mayor declared Mr Hill unanimously elected, and passed over to that gentleman the gold ring and chain, and handed him to the mayoral throne, amidst the plaudits of the council and the numerous citizens assembled in the hall.

"The Mayor elect said, he found some difficulty in giving expression to the complication of feelings arising in his bosom. If he was merely to acknowledge the great personal compliment conferred upon him by unanimously electing him to the highest official honour of the city, perhaps he might content himself with assuring the council that he felt deeply grateful for the honourable mark of esteem; but the warm and sincere expressions whirh accompanied the tender of the honour, not only rendered it greater, but increased his difficulty in expressing his sense of gratefulness. (Cheers.) And considerations of another character rose in rapid succession in his mind, for he was well aware that the office brought responsibility as well as dignity, and therefore he begged to add to his expressions of thanks, his deep sense of the responsibility he was undertaking, and to assure the council that his sincere actuating desire should be to maintain, unimpaired, the dignity of the office, and to pass to his successor unblemished the honours of this ancient mayoralty; for whether the duties devolving upon him had reference to the moral, social, or civil condition of the city, they should be discharged with fidelity, and all the ability he could command. Although with respect to much of the business he had not had that experience which gave ripened skill, he hoped to be enabled to conduct it unprejudiced and unbiassed by any party, or by any improper feeling; and it would be to him a source of heartfelt gratification if his exertions during his period of mayoralty won for him the thanks which were about to be accorded to his predecessor. The citizens might always calculate on his being alive to the interests of this ancient and loyal city—a city which would be associated with-his latest remembrances as the spot of those labours which led his friend Mr Harvey to mention his namely honourably in connexion with the cause of medical science and humanity. (Cheers.)"

From the *Lincolnshire Chronicle*, November 26, 1853.

" The Mayor's Dinner.—The most eloquent and important speech of the evening was delivered by Richard Mason, Esq., in reply to the toast of ' the Town Clerk.'—Mr Mason, after acknowledging the compliment paid to him, congratulated the citizens of Lincoln on the high character and attainments of their Chief-Magistrate. The late Mayor was known to the world for his attainments as an antiquarian and archæologist, sciences and pursuits which required great learning, deep research, and unwearied industry, and these qualifications their chief-magistrate possessed, as was well known, in an eminent degree. (Loud cheers.) Their present chief-magistrate would hand his name down to posterity as the originator of the ' non-restraint system' in

Lunatic Asylums,—a great onward movement in medical science, and a movement which had produced results for which every humane man felt deeply grateful. Our lunatics, since the discoveries of a Hill, were treated as human beings labouring under disease, instead of being regarded as raging brute beasts, to be kept in awe by horrid instruments of cruelty, and acts of ferocious barbarity. Mr Hill's claims to be considered the originator of the non-restraint system had been contested in the outset, but now the fact was fully established, and was recognized all over the kingdom, and indeed abroad also. In a Leader which appeared in the *Times* the other day, the fact was broadly stated; and in an edition of *Knight's Encyclopædia*, which he saw in Paris a short time ago, he read an article on insanity, from which he made the following extract :—

" ' Every part of the treatment of the insane has, of late years, been much modified by the introduction of a much milder mode of management. The total abolition of personal restraint, known as the *non-restraint system*, was first introduced at the Lincoln Asylum in 1837, and its complete success *there* led to its adoption at Hanwell in 1839, and shortly afterwards at Northampton, Gloucester, Lancaster, Stafford, and Glasgow. This system has since been adopted at the Haslar hospital, in France, &c.'

" The article then goes on to notice some mitigations of instrumental restraint which had taken place at the Bicêtre, in Paris, under Pinel, and continues:—

" ' But the declaration that mechanical restraints were never necessary, never justifiable, and always injurious, first made by Mr HILL, of Lincoln, has caused this march of improvement to proceed much more rapidly.' ' However opinions may differ as to the abolition of restraint in those Asylums which have not tried the experiment, we know that many thousands have been treated (since Mr Hill's suggestion) entirely without it, and in no Asylum where the new system has been introduced, has it been found necessary to abandon it ; that the reports of all these Asylums state their general condition to be improved, and the cures not to have decreased ; and, which we consider of equal importance, that the comfort of the incurables is most increased ; and we may, therefore, be justified in considering that within a few years the instruments of restraint now remaining will disappear, like those more severe ones which preceded them.'

" Mr Hill's claims had been contested because before he broached and carried into execution his ' non-restraint system,' improvements had been effected, and approaches to his system made. It was quite true that the treatment of the insane had been greatly ameliorated before Mr Hill carried into effect his system; but this no more invalidated his claim to be considered the originator of this system, than did the prior efforts of men who worked steam engines from collieries by cog and wheel invalidate the claim of a Stephenson to be deemed the inventor of the modern locomotive ; or the early discoveries in electricity to rob a Wheatstone of the merits of discovering the electric telegraph. Nearly every great discovery that was made was founded upon some preceding efforts which might seem to tend to the result ultimately achieved, and this was just the position which the worthy chief-magistrate occupied. (Loud cheers.) In the course of a few years, prejudice and calumny would be hushed, and Mr Hill's name, linked with the history of their country, would be recorded by the impartial pen of the historian as the name of one of the great benefactors of the human race. (Loud cheers.)"

(Appendix G.)

Cases of the two patients under treatment at the Lincoln Asylum during the period of the mitigation system; referred to in the Historical Sketch.

(*Case* 390.)

1832, *June* 18.—W. C., æt. 39, was admitted this day. He has been insane at times since the age of 17, and had a severe attack about three years ago, in consequence of being put to trouble for a small debt: the present attack came on about a fortnight ago, and he has, during the last five days, been in a state of considerable excitement: bowels confined: appetite good.

June 19. — W. C. is in a state of violent maniacal excitement, and cannot be persuaded to take any portion of his diet.

June 20.—W. B. and W. C. are refractory, and under restraint.

June 22.—W. C. continues violent and noisy; takes his food very irregularly, and in small quantities.

June 24.—W. C. no improvement, constantly throwing himself about, wears the muff to prevent him from tearing his clothes.

June 25.—W. C. has taken scarcely any portion of his breakfast; cannot be kept still, but is constantly throwing his head about, so as to render it impossible to feed him except by means of the feeder: had a pint-and-a-half of strong broth administered in this way at 3 p.m., and was fastened in bed by his hands and feet.

June 25.—W. C. had milk given him about 7 this evening by means of the feeder. 8½ p.m., dying on his back, pulse small and weak, respiration quick and labouring, excitement gone, bowels not moved since yesterday; passes his urine into the bed; feet warm; appears to have some tenderness about the epigastrium, but does not draw up his legs as if he suffered pain : he has had a small quantity of brandy and water administered, which appeared to arouse him a little. Appl. Cat. Sin. Cruribus et Empl. Canth. Nuch. Colli.— Continue the brandy and water at intervals if he can take it.

June 26. —W. C. continued lying in a state of exhaustion until about half-past one a.m., when he expired.

(*Case* 389.)

From June 17, 1832, to April 19, 1833.

1832, *June* 17.—S. L., aged 31, was admitted this day. He has been insane ten days; exciting cause, intemperance, &c.

June 19.—S. L. incoherent and rambling in his conversation.

June 20.—S. L. much excited, broke a window this morning, incoherent and singing very loudly.

June 21.—S. L. continues rambling and incoherent in his conversation : undressed himself this afternoon, and threw his clothes into the adjoining court, as he states, " *because the keepers had not done their duty in watching him ;*" no disposition to violence.

Tractable from this date to the 29th.

June 30 —S. L. not so well to-day, mischievous and tearing his clothes.

July 1.—S. L. is so high as to require moving to the noisy cell.

July 2.—S. L. destroyed his coat, waistcoat, and shirt in a few minutes *whilst the keeper was absent washing his braces;* he has worn the muff the rest of the day.

July 4.—S. L. very noisy and under restraint, to prevent him from tearing his clothes.

July 5.—S. L. noisy and violent, requiring seclusion the most of the day.

July 6.—S. L. is calmer to-day, and manageable without restraint.

July 7.—S. L. is excessively noisy, and secluded in the noisy cell.

July 8.—S. L. wild and incoherent; could not be kept in bed, and required fastening at bed-time by both hands.

July 9.—S. L. has been noisy most of the day, and required secluding in the noisy cell all the afternoon; at 6 this evening he became violent, and was put to bed after lying for some time on the floor of the cell.

July 10.—S. L. is very noisy, and required to be fastened to his bedstead.

July 11.—S. L. is still disposed to tear his clothes, and requires the constant use of the muff to prevent him; he passed a restless night, shouting and praying.

July 20.—S. L. is in a very excited state, requiring the muff; he has been very violent for several days.

July 21.—S. L. so violent as to require fastening in the chair as well by his feet as by his hands and body; shouting and singing all the afternoon and evening.

July 22.—S. L. was confined all the morning in a chair in the noisy cell: *the handlocks were removed at dinner, one of them having become twisted so as to make pressure on the hand;* at night he was very violent, and *on examining his elbow and fore-arm, I find it much inflamed and swollen.* Appl. Hirudines xviij et postea Cat. Panis.

July 23.—S. L. refuses his diet: he had about one hour's sleep during last night; this morning *the arm is greatly swollen and soft to the touch ;* there is less heat and tension of the skin than last night. Cont. Cat.—to-night the arm is much reduced in size.

July 24.—S. L. steadily refuses food—arm quite well.

July 24.—S. L. refused all nourishment—forcibly fed twice to-day.

July 26.—S. L. fed twice: during the morning he was kept in bed without difficulty, but in the afternoon the same means were necessary as used yesterday.

July 27.—S. L. no sustenance except by forcible administration—diarrhœa.

July 27.—S. L. food and medicine administered by force. No evacuation since morning.

July 28.—S. L. diarrhœa returned about half-past three this afternoon. Colour leaving the cheeks, food administered forcibly.

July 29.—S. L. no diarrhœa to-day ; pulse 110 and quick ; frequent desire for cold water ; takes his medicine, but requires his food administering by force: slept well last night.

July 30.—S. L. one copious evacuation in the night and several to-day ; pulse 100 and firm: takes no sustenance except by means of the feeder: rested well during last night: although conscious of what is passing, he lies in a state of apparent insensibility both day and night.

July 31.—S. L. has not required feeding to day : he ate a hearty dinner; a great change for the better has taken place since yesterday. He sat up in the gentlemen's room, and was taken to the centre house to sleep.

Aug. 1.—S. L's. bowels continue lax : he is so dirty as to require removing to the North Gallery.

Aug. 3 and 4.—S. L.—insensible to natural calls.

Aug. 7.—S. L. has broken several articles of furniture, and cannot be left for a moment.

Aug. 10.—S. L. appeared excited this morning, although

at present he does not speak : at bed-time he was found walking about his room, and would not lie in bed ; he is menacing, and disposed to strike those about him, requiring to be fastened by one hand to his bedstead.

Aug. 11.—-S. L. could not be kept in bed without fastening last night ; to-day he is violent and under restraint.

Aug. 12.—S. L. is violent, and required restraint all day ; he required fastening in one of the tub-bedsteads of the North Gallery.

Aug. 13.—S. L. refuses all sustenance to-day, and requires feeding by force ; could not be kept in bed last night except by means of a tub-bedstead, to which he was fastened by his hands and feet : to-day he was rolling on the floor of the gallery.

Aug. 14.—S. L. has had nourishment administered twice to-day by means of the feeder; still disposed to throw himself about the floor, and cannot be kept in a chair.

Aug. 17.—S. L. forcibly fed.

Aug. 22.—S. L. broke one of the windows this after-noon.

Aug. 25.—S. L.: THE BOOT HOBBLES INVENTED BY Dr CHARLESWORTH FOR CONFINING THE FEET TO THE BEDSTEAD were applied this evening, and on looking at the patient at bed-time 10 P.M. I find the ancles free from pressure, and the object of the instrument completely answered.

Aug. 26.—S. L. quiet, and not requiring restraint during the day.

Sept. 3.—S. L. became violent, and struck his keeper: *two or three attendants were required to secure him.*

Sept. 4.—S. L. continues talkative: refused his dinner, and is prone to violence, if not under restraint.

Sept. 5.—S. L. so violent as to require his removal to the North Gallery.

Sept. 6. S. L. violent and unmanageable: it is necessary for him to remain in the North Gallery.

Sept. 8.—S. L. is getting more mischievous, and tearing his clothes; constantly muttering to himself: he cannot be trusted without restraint.

Sept. 9.—S. L. has again become mischievous and violent, tore his coat and shirt: generally rolling on the floor.

Sept. 11.—S. L. bruised his right ear this morning by throwing himself against the bedstead; has torn his clothes very much.

Sept. 12.—S. L. has a carbuncle forming on the back. Fiat incisio cruciformis tumoris and applic. Cataplasm.

Sept. 14.—S. L. abscess on the scalp opened this evening.

Sept. 17.—S. L. still bent on mischief, and under restraint.

Sept. 20.—S. L. cannot be trusted for a minute without restraint—constant disposition to tear his clothes; requires fastening in bed by his hands and feet.

Sept. 23.—S. L. is rather better to-day, and has been allowed to be without restraint.

Sept. 30.—S. L. does not require restraint, but still much inclined for mischief—his keeper cannot leave him for a moment.

Oct. 3.—S. L. under restraint.

Oct. 11.—No improvement, if anything more disposed to mischief.

Oct. 15.—S. L. has a small swelling on the occiput, with unhealthy inflammation surrounding it, which is tender on being touched. Appl. Cat. Lini. mane nocteque.

Oct. 18.—S. L. high, and at times violent.

Oct. 19.—S. L. has been exceedingly violent and unmanageable all day, throwing himself on the ground, and trying to escape from his keeper, who sometimes requires assistance.

Oct. 20.—S. L. is gradually getting worse

Oct. 21.—S. L. violent and unmanageable.

Oct. 22.—S. L. cannot have stockings kept on his feet—so violent as to require three of the keepers to dress him—is becoming dirty in his habits.

Oct. 23.—S. L. continues as yesterday. To have his allowance of meat withdrawn and pudding substituted in its place—the same difficulty occurred in dressing him this morning.

Oct. 24.—S. L. continues violent, and bruising his feet by kicking against his chair.

Oct. 25.—S. L. violent, and *constantly kicking his heels against the chair in which he is fastened;* to prevent further injury to his heels he was placed in bed until a cushion can be made for the front of his chair. 11 p.m., more violent, and *chafing his arms against the sides of his bedstead so as to erode the skin. The* WAISTCOAT *has just been put on,* as the *mildest and most efficient mode of restraint in these particular cases.*

Oct. 26.—S. L. *had the waistcoat on last night and the whole of to-day*—this evening he is throwing his head about in a violent manner—no disposition to sleep—pupils rather dilated—cannot be left for a minute.

Oct. 27.—S. L., by constantly throwing up his arms during the night, loosened the waistcoat sufficiently to get it off—the keeper in attendance had occasion to call up another to assist him in replacing the waistcoat—he has been throwing his head about the most of the night.

Oct. 28.—S. L. enjoyed some sleep during the night—continues to throw his head about in a violent manner at intervals.

Oct. 29.—S. L. had some sleep during the night—has been calm all day, and not requiring restraint.

Oct. 31.—S. L. had a quiet night—he is exceedingly mischievous this morning, and inclined to tear his clothes, and can only be restrained from doing so by the muff.

Nov. 1.—S. L's. ear very much enlarged, poultice applied to it—he is *constantly under restraint* from his disposition to mischief.

Nov. 2.—S. L. had a motion during the night, and covered himself from head to foot with fæces. Ear still much enlarged. Cont. Cat. Panis. There are some papulæ about the lower extremities.

Nov. 3.—S. L. had a motion in bed—he requires restraint to prevent him tearing his clothes.

Nov. 4.—S. L.. The ear, which was emptied of a large. quantity of pus and serum, has filled again since last night.

Nov. 5.—S. L. Ear again filled with sero-purulent fluid. Cont. Cataplasm.

Nov. 6.—S. L. Abscess filled with pus.

Nov. 7.—S. L. No change in the state of his mind. Ear distended with pus.

Nov. 8.—S. L. had an evacuation during the night, and covered himself with fæces. Ear as yesterday.

Nov. 9.—S. L. covered himself with fæculent matter. Ear not quite so distended as yesterday—calmer.

Nov. 10.—S. L. Ear continues to discharge a considerable quantity of pus when opened. Appetite good—continues to require restraint.

Nov. 11.—S. L. has several sores upon his lower extremities, which he scratches at night, causing them to bleed—becoming dirty in the day as well as at night.

Nov. 16.—S. L. Several of the sores are healing—has a sore on his right heel, to which a poultice is applied—it was brought on by his habit of kicking the chair, to which a cushion has since been fitted.

Nov. 17.—S. L. Abscess of the ear is beginning to contract—there is still considerable thickening of the parts, and some discharge, but not to any great extent—general health better—sores healing fast.

316

Nov. 18.—S. L. has had a trial made of a petticoat, on account of his constantly wetting himself, causing excoriation.

Nov. 20.—S. L. continues dirty and wet in his habits.

Nov. 23.—S. L. was eating his fæces this morning when the keeper entered his room.

Nov. 27.—S. L. Sores healing.

Nov. 29.—S. L. Abscess in the ear discharges again to a considerable extent.

Dec. 2.—S. L. is violent and unmanageable this morning; he could not be dressed until two additional keepers came to assist his own attendant.

Dec. 6.—S. L. Sores on his legs nearly well.

Dec. 7.—S. L. Abscess of the ear nearly well, in other respects no change.

Dec. 13.—S. L. is calmer and more easily managed than he has been of late—*is led about by the keeper every day*—most of the sores healed.

Dec. 14.—S. L. is more manageable, and walking in the gallery—*he is not able to be trusted without restraint.*

Dec. 15.—S. L. is considerably calmer than of late, and is able to take moderate exercise in the gallery—his habits are less dirty, and his general appearance improved.

Dec. 16.—S. L. quieter, and able to wear his trowsers, which he has not done for the past month—he is without restraint.

Dec. 17.—S. L. *is not so calm, and cannot be trusted without restraint.*

Dec. 18.—S. L. continues as yesterday.

Dec. 19.—S. L. is becoming dirty again, and requires the petticoat to prevent excoriation.

Dec. 20.—S L. *cannot be trusted at liberty*, though he is quieter than he generally is.

Dec. 21.—S. L. No improvement—dirty, and cannot wear his trowsers—seldom speaks to any one.

Dec. 22 —S. L. is still wet and dirty—does not converse at all.

Dec. 23.—S. L. very dirty this morning; face flushed, appetite good, rests quietly at night, is sullen, and does not notice any one.

Dec. 24.—S. L. sullen, and does not answer questions; is very dirty in his person.

Dec. 27.—S. L. is much more excited, and *requiring the Belt.*

Dec. 30.—S. L. was not fastened last night, as a trial, but contrived to cover himself with fæces before morning—the walls of his room were also in a filthy state.

1833, *Jan.* 1.—S. L. has a wound across the root of the penis which appears to have been inflicted with a sharp body—on examining his person nothing has been discovered upon him, nor any of those patients about him—*his straw bed* has also been examined without anything being found by which the patient could have injured himself.

Jan. 2.—S. L. very dirty in bed-room—wound going on well—*he is quite imbecile, and takes no cognizance of what passes around him.*

Jan. 5.—S. L. *The keeper is leading this patient about the gallery*—there is not any change in the condition of this patient since last report, nor is he in any way improved.

Jan. 8.—S. L. continues to be wet and dirty in his habits.

Jan. 9.—S. L. is again becoming more dirty—*he is not at all violent, but sits the whole day in a state of childishness,* without opening his lips to speak to any one.

Jan. 10.—S. L. is as reported yesterday.

Jan. 11.—S. L. is still in a very dirty state, and requires the petticoat.

Jan. 12.—S. L. is mischievous, and in no way improved.

Jan. 14.—S. L. quiet but not improved—does not speak or converse with any one.

Jan. 15.—S. L. is mischievous, and trying to undress himself.

Jan. 16.—S. L. is mischievous, *requiring the Belt.*

Jan. 17.—S. L. dirty and mischievous, requires the Belt.

Jan. 21.—S. L. is mischievous and dirty.

Jan. 24.—S. L. No improvement, does not speak to any one.

Jan. 25.—S. L. quiet, and not requiring restraint.

Jan. 31.—S. L. rather cleaner, and has had his trowsers put on instead of the petticoat.

Feb. 16.—S. L. seems more inclined to mischief.

Feb. 17.—S. L. does not improve, seldom speaks, and is in *a childish state.*

Feb. 21.—S. L is not changed—he did not dirt his bed last night—in the day he is wet and dirty, and continues to wear the petticoat.

Feb. 28.—S. L. has a sore on his left leg, which he is in the habit of scratching.

March 7.—S. L. lay quietly last night without being fastened—he threw the fæces passed in the night upon the wall and bedstead, as well as the floor of his bed room.

March 16.—S. L. *made so much noise in his room last night that it will be necessary to secure him again by his hands and feet* to prevent him getting out of bed.

April 19.—S. L. does not vary—*he has been calm for a considerable period, but is as dirty as ever.*

REYNELL AND WEIGHT, Printers, Little Pulteney-street, Haymarket.

ERRATA.

Page 159, note, line 1, for "lectures" read "lecture."
Page 198, line 15, for "carry" read "carrying."